Medicolegal Essentials in Healthcare

Edited by

Jason Payne-James FRCS LL.M MB MAE (Edin & Eng)
Forensic Physician, London;
Honorary Senior Research Fellow, Department of Gastroenterology & Nutrition,
Central Middlesex Hospital, London, UK

Peter Dean LL.M MB BS BDS (Hons) DRCOG
H.M. Coroner, Essex No 2 District;
Forensic Physician, London, UK

Ian Wall LL.M BA MB BS DCH DRCOG MRCGP Barrister at Law
Forensic Physician, London, UK

CHURCHILL LIVINGSTONE
NEW YORK EDINBURGH LONDON MADRID MELBOURNE SAN FRANCISCO AND TOKYO 1996

CHURCHILL LIVINGSTONE
CHURCHILL LIVINGSTONE
Medical Division of Pearson Professional Limited

Distributed in the United States of America by Churchill
Livingstone Inc., 650 Avenue of the Americas, New York, N.Y.
10011, and by associated companies, branches and
representatives throughout the world.

First Published 1996

ISBN 0443 052409

British Library Cataloguing in Publication Data
A catalogue record for this book is available from the British
Library.

Library of Congress Cataloging in Publication Data
A catalogue record for this book is available from the Library
of Congress.

Medical Knowledge is constantly changing. As new
information becomes available, changes in treatment,
procedures, equipment and the use of drugs become necessary.
The editors/authors/contributors and the publishers have, as
far as it is possible, taken care to ensure that the information
given in this text is accurate and up to date. However, readers
are strongly advised to confirm that the information, especially with regard to drug usage, complies with the latest legislation and standards of practice.

Produced through Longman Malaysia, PP

Medicolegal Essentials in Healthcare

Books are to be ret⸱   ⸱ore
the last dat⸱

For Churchill Livingstone

Commissioning Editor: Gavin Smith
Copy Editor: Alison Bowers
Project Controller: Anita Sekhri
Cover Design: Keith Kale

Contents

The contents of this book follow the Interpretation Act 1978, so in that unless specifically stated otherwise, words importing the masculine gender include the feminine and words importing the feminine gender include the masculine.

Contributors

Anthony Barton MA MB BS
Solicitor and Medical Practitioner

Diana Brahams
Barrister at Law
Old Square Chambers, London, UK

Peter Dean LL.M MB BS BDS (Hons) DRCOG
HM Coroner, Essex No 2 District;
Forensic Physician, London, UK

Alain Gregoire MB BS DRCOG MRCPsych
Consultant Psychiatrist, Salisbury Healthcare;
Honorary Senior Lecturer in Psychiatry,
Southampton University, Southampton, UK

Ivor H Harrison MPharm PhD FRPharmS MBIRA (Hons)
Senior Lecturer in Pharmacy Law, Welsh School of Pharmacy,
Cardiff, Wales, UK

Catherine E James MB ChB FRCOG
Medicolegal Adviser, Medical Defence Union, London, UK

Gill Korgaonkar LL.B LL.M
Director of studies and Principal Lecturer in Law,
Division of Law, University of Hertfordshire, UK

Allan Levy QC LL.B
Barrister Specialising in Child Law and Medical Law, London,
UK

Robert Parker MSc
Homograft Department Manager, Royal Brompton Hospital,
London, UK

Simon D. W. Payne LL.M MB BS FRCS (Ed) FRCS (Eng) FFAEM
Consultant in Accident and Emergency Surgery,
The Royal Hampshire County Hospital, Winchester, UK

Jason Payne-James LL.M MB FRCS (Edin & Eng)
Forensic Physician; Honorary Senior Research Fellow,
Department of Gastroenterology and Nutrition, Central Middlesex
Hospital, London, UK

Christobel Saunders MB BS FRCS
Lecturer, The Breast Unit, Guys and St Thomas Hospital, London,
UK

Peter Schutte MB ChB MRCGP DMJ
Deputy Head of Advisory Services, Medical Defence Union,
London, UK

John Skone LL.M MD FFPHM
Formerly Chief Administrative Medical Officer and Director of
Public Health Medicine, South Glamorgan Health Authority, UK

Pauline Smith RGN RSCN BA (Hons) BSc
Nurse Teacher, Health Authority, London, UK

Diana M R Tribe LL.B MA
Head of School and Law, University of Hertfordshire; Victory
Research Fellow, Institute of Advanced Legal Studies, University
of London, UK

Ian Wall LL.M BA MB BS DCH DROG MRCGP
Barrister at Law, Forensic Physician, London, UK

Foreword

We live in an increasingly complicated world and it becomes more and more difficult to know where to seek the answers to problems which affect so many of us. One area of particular importance is healthcare. Whether medical practitioner, nurse or other health professional, administrator or patient and patient's family, nowadays there appears to be less willingness to accept decisions and far greater opportunities for disputes to arise and quicker recourse to litigation.

This invaluable book, with chapters written by a wide variety of distinguished contributors, cover a vast number of important subjects. It ranges across the procedures of courts, civil and criminal, disciplinary bodies including the General Medical Council and complaints procedures in the National Health Service to important and controversial subjects such as euthanasia, organ donation, abortion and reproductive health, ethical and practical considerations of clinical trials. There are chapters on the Children Act, medical negligence, consent to medical treatment and confidentiality. The role of the coroner is explained in detail.

The co-editors are particularly well qualified from their own medical and legal training and experience to assemble a fascinating and comprehensive collection of the medicolegal aspects of life from birth to death. It should be in the bookcase of every health professional but would seem to me to be equally invaluable to the lawyer and to many members of the public.

The Rt Hon Lady Justice Butler-Sloss DBE
Royal Courts of Justice, London

Editors' Note

The aim of this book is to provide an overview of those legal issues
most relevant to individuals working in the healthcare professions.
The need for a basic understanding of the legal framework in
which healthcare is provided, and of the role that law and the judiciary play in the working lives of all such professionals, is now
being recognised by the increasing emphasis placed on the teaching of legal and ethical principles to undergraduate students in
medicine, nursing, pharmacy and allied professions. Knowledge of
these subjects has become an intrinsic part of many teaching courses, and there is no part of the wide spectrum of healthcare provision that does not, at some time, require an understanding and
consideration of these basic medicolegal principles. Those professionals already qualified and in practice, both in hospitals and the
community, regularly experience the need to have appropriate
knowledge of many of these issues. With increasing frequency
items of medicolegal significance appear in the news and media.
This book looks at those areas where law and medicine commonly
meet. The chapters are written by a multidisciplinary group of
practitioners with special interest or experience in their subjects.
We hope that these medicolegal essentials will provide a sound
basis for undergraduates, postgraduates and all healthcare
providers, and will inspire some to develop, further their own
interest, knowledge and understanding of the growing and increasingly important interface between medicine and the law.

The law in this book is stated as of April 1 1996

JP-J, PD, IW   London 1996

Table of Cases

Table of Statutes

Statutory Instruments (SI) are rules made by Ministers of the Crown pursuant to powers conferred on them due to provisions contains in the relevant Act of Parliament.

1. The courts and legal procedure

Ian Wall, Jason Payne-James, Peter Dean

Few areas of healthcare practice in the United Kingdom are untouched by the law. The purpose of this chapter is to provide a broad outline of the legal system in England and Wales, in order to facilitate an understanding of the subject matter of subsequent chapters. Scotland enjoys both its own set of laws and its own hierarchy of civil and criminal courts. Though distinct, Scottish law has many similarities to that across the border, Westminster being the ultimate legislative body and the House of Lords the ultimate appellate court.

THE LAW

Laws are rules that govern orderly behaviour in a collective society. In England and Wales the main sources of these laws are Parliament and the courts of law.

Parliamentary law

Parliament is the principal organ of legislation in the United Kingdom. It is composed of the House of Commons, the House of Lords and the Monarch. Parliament is in theory omnicompetent, and under the doctrine of the 'Sovereignty of Parliament', laws made by it cannot be altered by the courts. Parliamentary legislation is known as primary legislation.

Prospective Parliamentary legislation begins life as a political policy. The Government of the day may consult interested parties before publishing a broad discussion document on the issue, called a Green Paper. Following further scrutiny a White Paper will be published which represents a finer statement on policy. A Bill will then be drafted based on information thus collected, and presented before the House of Commons. The Bill, in the course of its enactment, will undergo a number of readings, followed by detailed analysis of its provisions in a Committee stage. The Bill is read again to the House, and if acceptable will then be passed to the House of Lords to undergo a similar process of scrutiny, prior to being sent to the Monarch for Royal Assent. Having successfully negotiated this path the Bill then becomes an Act of Parliament, or Statute. A prospective statute may also *mutatis mutandis* ('the necessary changes being made for context') commence in, and pass through, the House of Lords.

The passage of primary legislation is a relatively open exercise where external public pressure has the potential to influence the final outcome. This method of legislation, however, is time-consuming and too inflexible to meet the needs of rapidly changing situations.

Delegated legislation

It would be impractical, if not impossible, for Parliament to pass detailed legislation in an attempt to cover all spheres of human activity. Parliamentary legislation therefore often contains provisions empowering Ministers, governmental departments and inferior administrative bodies to make regulations which have the force of law, in order to facilitate the detailed logistical exercise of executing and administering Parliamentary wishes. These laws are known as secondary or delegated legislation. This process is less open to public scrutiny, though it has the advantage of affording a greater degree of flexibility in its response to differing, and rapidly changing, circumstance.

Much of the running of the National Health Service is based on delegated legislation. Responsibility for providing and administering the service rests on the Secretary of State for Health acting pursuant to enabling acts of Parliament. The Secretary of State is a cabinet minister and is head of the Department of Health, being assisted by a Minister of Health. It is the duty of the Secretary of State to ensure that the legislative wishes of Parliament are executed. The Department of Health will further delegate certain administrative functions to the various administrative tiers within the service, and seek to ensure compliance with Acts of Parliament or governmental policy by means of circulars and executive letters. Both the Secretary of State and these inferior administrative bodies exercise wide discretionary powers in pursuit of their duties, such as in the allocation and management of resources.

Control of administrative powers in the NHS

Ministerial responsibility

Ministers of Health, in common with other government ministers, may be required to answer questions in Parliament on both their actions and those of their department. Most matters can be, and indeed often are, dealt with by way of written replies. Open questions from the floor of Parliament may be the source of considerable political embarrassment, and unwelcome media and public attention.

Parliamentary review

The provision of health care may come under scrutiny from Parliamentary Select Committees composed of Members of Parliament who will have a special interest, and therefore knowledge, of a particular field. They have wide powers to examine documents and summon persons before them in pursuance of their duties. There are two Select Committees concerned with health matters; the Select Committee on Health and the Select Committee for Administration, which examines reports from the Ombudsman.

The Ombudsman

The Health Service Commissioner or Ombudsman is charged by Parliament with the investigation of complaints concerning maladministration within the Health Service. Complainants are able to approach the Ombudsman directly provided the matter has been brought to the attention of the Health Authority first. The Ombudsman has no powers to examine complaints of errors in clinical judgments or complaints against General Practitioners.

Judicial review

The High Court maintains an inherent jurisdiction, through judicial review, to supervise administrative bodies to ensure that they do not usurp the sovereign will of Parliament. The doctrine of *ultra vires* (literally 'beyond power — used to describe any acts that are in excess of authority conferred by law) exists to ensure that administrative bodies act within the spirit as well as the letter of the law, that they exercise their powers 'reasonably',[a] legally, in good faith and for proper purposes. In policing the exercise of discretionary powers the courts will wish to balance the need to protect the citizen with the need to ensure an efficient executive.

The courts are however unwilling to substitute their own judgment for the 'reasonable' judgment of those who are responsible for the allocation of resources. In R v Cambridge DHA ex parte B[1] the court, though sympathetic to the plight of the applicant, a child with leukaemia, upheld the Health Authority's decision not to allocate resources to treat due to the grim prognosis of the disease. In R v North West Thames RHA ex parte Daniels[2], the Health Authority, as part of a rationalisation of resources, had closed down a bone marrow unit which would have been able to provide the appropriate treatment care for the applicant, a child with a rare metabolic disease. The courts found that although the Authority had technically acted illegally by breaching an NHS regulation requiring them to consult before deciding on closure; they did not, however, order the Authority to establish a similar unit at a nearby hospital.

Leave for an application for judicial review[b] will only be permitted by the courts in cases which raise 'public law' issues, and only then when the aggrieved has sufficient interest in the outcome of the case (known as locus standi).[c] The process of judicial review only allows the 'supervising' court to invalidate an illegal decision, and send it back to the original deciding body for reconsideration. The supervising court cannot substitute its own opinion on the substantive merits of the decision, and in this important aspect judicial review differs from appeal.

Tribunals

Tribunals perform an appellate role (hear appeals) controlling the proper exercise of discretionary administrative powers by administrative offices or persons. One example is the Mental Health Review Tribunal which hears appeals from those aggrieved by decisions on compulsory committal or detention in psychiatric institutions. Tribunals have the benefit of being flexible and cheap, and

---

1 R v Cambridge District Health Authority ex parte B The Times 15 March 1995
2 R v North West Thames Regional Health Authority ex parte Daniels The Times 22 June 1993

usually possess specialist expertise in their narrow fields. There exists a statutory route of appeal to the Divisional Court (see below) from a decision made by a tribunal tainted by an error of law.

JUDICIAL LAW

The other main source of law is 'judge made' law resulting from decisions in the courts. Consistency and fairness in judicial law are maintained to a certain extent by the 'doctrine of precedent' which ensures that the principles enunciated in one court will normally be followed subsequently by both courts of similar standing and inferior courts. The House of Lords, by way of exception, is not so bound and has jurisdiction to overrule its previous decisions. The courts will always be bound by the provisions of statutory law, though they have a role in construing or interpreting the language of statutes (and therefore sometimes their substantive intent).

Branches of law

The law is divided into a number of specialist fields, each with its own rules. The two main categories that are of relevance in the healthcare field are civil law, and to a lesser extent, criminal law. Civil law is concerned with the resolution of disputes between individuals, and it is the aggrieved party who undertakes the action. Criminal law is concerned with offences whose nature is of sufficient importance that the state undertakes their prosecution. The substantive rules of evidence and procedure differ between civil and criminal jurisdictions, as do the penalties.[d] The courts are also similarly split into civil and criminal jurisdiction, which means that civil cases are heard in one type of court and criminal cases in another, the courts of each jurisdiction being arranged in an hierarchical manner.

The Civil Courts

The magistrates' court is the lowest of the civil courts in England and Wales, and has a limited role in civil disputes. Above the magistrates' court is the County Court. In the presence of a circuit judge the County Courts will hear up to 90% of all civil disputes each year.

The High Court has unlimited jurisdiction in civil cases, but for most types of proceedings it shares jurisdiction with the County Courts. The High Court itself comprises three divisions: the Chancery Division, which specialises in matters of company law, trusts etc.; the Family Division, specialising in matrimonial issues and matters relating to minors; and the Queen's Bench Division, which deals with general civil matters. It is usual for judges in the High Court to sit in the absence of a jury. The High Court has a number of provincial offices known as district registries, and along with the Crown Court is part of the Supreme Court of Judicature of England and Wales. The Queen's Bench Division sits as a divisional court to hear appeals from magistrates' courts (on civil matters) and tribunals. The Civil Division of the Court of Appeal will hear appeals from the High Court and the County Courts, and is presided over by the Master of the Rolls and the Lords Justices of Appeal. The ultimate appellate court for England and Wales, Scotland and Northern Ireland is the House of Lords[e]. Questions arising before an English court, concerning the interpretation or validity of any act of the institutions of the European Community, may be referred to the European Court of Justice for a ruling, if such a ruling is necessary for the English court to reach its judgment.

The Criminal Courts

The magistrates' courts play a much more important role in criminal cases, and the vast majority of criminal cases will appear before the magistrates either for trial or committal. The magistrates will try and sentence minor or summary criminal offences, while the Crown Court hears the more serious offences. Appeals from the Crown Court are made to the Criminal Division of the Court of Appeal, and thence to the House of Lords on important points of law.

Criminal procedure

The initial stage of criminal procedure is usually arrest by police, which along with the subsequent conduct of the detention is governed by the Police and Criminal Evidence Act 1984.[f] Since the Prosecution of Offences Act 1985 the prosecution of offenders has been undertaken by a centralised body known as the Crown Prosecution Service (CPS) headed by the Director of Public Prosecutions. The decision of the CPS as to whether it will prosecute a case is based on the public interest, and if there is a likelihood of a conviction.

Preliminary hearings

With few exceptions all criminal cases involving indictable offences will appear before the magistrates prior to the Crown Court. The purpose of this preliminary hearing is to act as a filter and assess whether there is a *prima facie* (literally 'on first appearance' — used to describe cases in which there is some support for the allegation made) case for the defendant to answer at Crown Court.

Civil procedure

Prior to initiating formal legal proceedings an aggrieved party may take advantage of a number of informal avenues, such as a complaint to the relevant Health Authority or the Family Health Service Authority (FHSA) if the complaint is against a general practitioner, or to the General Medical Council (GMC). The aggrieved's decision to institute formal proceedings may be helped by speaking to the Citizens' Advice Bureau or a support organisation such as the Association for the Victims of Medical Accidents (AVMA), who may be able to put him or her in contact with a solicitor experienced in such matters.

The basis of the civil system is to settle disputes between individuals, and to compensate the aggrieved, usually in financial terms. Cases involving personal injury that result from medical negligence are dealt with by the civil courts, unless there is evidence of 'gross' negligence, in which case the CPS may decide to pursue a criminal conviction.

Civil actions are commenced by the aggrieved party (the plaintiff), usually via a solicitor. Prior to the formal issuance of proceedings, the plaintiff's solicitor will usually inform the other party of the intention to commence an action. This will enable a dialogue to be opened in which it may be possible to resolve a claim by negotiation without costly recourse to the courts.

The procedure for pursuing a claim throughout the civil courts is governed by the Rules of the Supreme Court (RSC). As an example an action for negligence or personal injury is formally commenced by the plaintiff filling in and issuing a standard legal document known as a writ, in either the High Court or the County Court.[g]

On the writ, the plaintiff will state the nature of his claim and the relief sought (i.e. damages). The writ will be issued by the court sealing it, and it will then be served on the defendant usually with a medical report outlining the injuries complained of. The defendant will then acknowledge its service and indicate an intention to defend the action or not. If there is an intention to defend, there then follows a predetermined sequence of events in which the parties, through their legal representatives, state the facts of their respective sides of the dispute in stylised legally drafted documents called *pleadings*, the role of which is to clarify the substance of the issues between the parties prior to putting them before the court.

Discovery

Parties to an action often possess documents, the contents of which may be relevant to the case in hand. Discovery is the name given to the procedure whereby one of the parties in litigation discloses the existence of such documents to the other, and later offers them up for physical inspection. In a High Court action for personal injuries a party who intends to rely on expert evidence is required to disclose the substance of such evidence to the other party in the form of a written report (RSC Ord 25, r 8 (1)(b)). Discovery usually takes place after the close of pleadings, though in cases of personal injury where only by the inspection of relevant medical records will the plaintiff be aware of the existence of cause of action, the rules provide for pre-action discovery (Supreme Court Act 1981, s33(2)).

Individuals have a legal right of access to information contained in their medical records subsequent to 1st November 1991 under the Access to Health Records Act 1990. Section 33(2) will still be relevant, however, for records made prior to that date, though somewhat illogically there is no such time limit for notes held on computer.[h]

Future advances

Civil procedure in the United Kingdom has been criticised for being time-consuming, expensive and unfair. Recommendations have been made to streamline and hasten civil procedure and limit the duration of court hearings, but these have not as yet been instigated.

REFERENCES

a   This is the so-called test of 'Wednesbury unreasonableness' (*Associated Provincial Picture Houses* v *Wednesbury Corporation* [1948] 1 KB 223). It has a number of formulations. In essence, a court will only intervene if a decision taken is one which no reasonable body could have arrived at if it had been taking into account all relevant matters, or it is a decision that is so wrong that no reasonable person could have sensibly taken that view

b   Applications for judicial reviews are written in the form *R* v *A ex p B*. *R* (the Monarch) v *A* (the respondent; the body whose decision is the subject of the action) *ex parte* (on behalf of) *B* (the aggrieved party). The Rules of the Supreme Court Order 53 describe the procedure for applying for judicial review

c   This concept is employed to limit the unnecessary hindrance of public bodies in the exercise of their functions by vexatious litigants, or pressure groups

d   There will often be roughly corresponding offences in civil and criminal jurisdictions, for example assault in criminal law and trespass in civil law. Criminal actions will take precedence but this does not preclude an individual from taking a separate private civil action for damages under the corresponding civil offence

e   The Judicial Committee of the Privy Council is the ultimate appellate court for the Isle of Man, the Channel Islands and the various UK dependencies. It also hears appeals from the General Medical Council, and certain other tribunals

f   This came into force in 1986. Revised codes were introduced in 1995 to implement changes in the law brought about by the Criminal Justice and Public Order Act 1994

g   Cases of personal injury involving claims less than £50 000 must be commenced in the County Courts; High Court and County Court Jurisdiction Order, Art. 5

h   Data Protection (Subject Access Modification) (Health) Order 1987, pursuant to the Data Protection Act 1984

FURTHER READING

Administrative Law:
Wade H W R, Forsythe C 1994 Administrative law. Clarendon Press, Oxford

Constitutional Law:
Brazier R, De Smith S A 1989 Constitutional and administrative law. Penguin, London

Criminal Procedure:
Sprack J (ed) 1992 Emmins on criminal procedure, 5th edn. Blackstone Press, London

Civil Procedure
Hare J O, Hill R N 1991 Civil litigation. Longman, London
Police and Criminal Evidence Act 1984, 1985, 1992, 1995: Codes of Practice. HMSO, London

2. Professional bodies and discipline

Jason Payne-James, Pauline Smith

INTRODUCTION

Regulation of standards of different healthcare professions varies widely. Some professions have disciplinary procedures that are governed by statute, and others by codes of practice or guidelines set by bodies established for that purpose alone, or by bodies supervising or giving advice on a whole range of issues, such as negotiating for pay and conditions, or supervising undergraduate and postgraduate education.

The majority of these bodies have a role in setting or defining standards of practice and providing the means by which practitioners who are deemed to have failed to achieve such standards can be disciplined. They are thus the key source of accountability for a practitioner within his or her profession. Sanctions vary dependent on the regulating body, and may for example allow for the removal of a practitioner from a register (which in certain cases may render the individual unable to practise and thus deprive him or her of a livelihood), or for the supervision of that practitioner when working, or may make requirements for retraining. The Professions Supplementary to Medicine Act 1960 provides a statutory framework throughout the UK for the registration, training, professional conduct and discipline of a number of healthcare professions. These are chiropodists; dietitians; medical laboratory scientific officers; occupational therapists; orthoptists; physiotherapists and radiographers. This accounts for a total of 90 000 registered practitioners. The Act created the Council for the Professions Supplementary to Medicine (CPSM) which coordinates the work of the Boards responsible for each profession. The Council has 23 members — one for each profession; of the others, six are doctors (six nominated by medical organisations). Four persons, of whom only two may be doctors and none can belong to a profession regulated by the Act, are appointed jointly by Secretaries of State. Five others are appointed by the Privy Council. None may belong to any of the professions or be doctors. Currently the Act is subject to a review, the terms of reference of which are: 'To review the role, functions and organisation of the statutory bodies established under the Professions Supplementary to Medicine Act 1960 so as to ensure that they are adequately accountable to Parliament for the exercise of their statutory functions, and that they operate efficiently, effectively and economically.'

In particular the review will examine the structure and constitution, interrelationships, functions and policy objectives of each body, and its relationship with Government, employers, educational institutions, professional organisations and the public; and examine the scope for improvements in the way the statutory bodies plan and control their activities so as to secure value for money.

The amount of 'self-regulation' of professional bodies is an area of great concern to many, as it is often perceived that the professional body acts in the interest of its members rather than the interests of the patients, clients or consumers. However it is accepted by many that 'self-regulation' is a satisfactory means of control, whereby the regulatory mechanism is controlled by the profession itself, is backed by statute and is financially independent of the state. In the UK, government support for 'self-regulation' has been reaffirmed by the passing of the Osteopaths Act 1993, which created the General Osteopathic Council. The Act provides for the Council to be the single, statutory, self-governing, regulatory body for osteopathy, able to enforce a strict code of professional conduct, to ensure that all practitioners are trained to the same high standards of clinical expertise and competence and to provide patients with all the necessary safeguards. The Council was appointed in 1996 and will draw up rules and regulations for approval by the Privy Council in 1997.

The constitution and functions of two bodies — the General Medical Council[a] (for doctors) and the United Kingdom Central Committee (for nurses) — will be considered in more detail.

THE GENERAL MEDICAL COUNCIL

The General Medical Council (GMC) was first established by statute by the Medical Act 1858 and consisted of a membership of 24, all of whom were medically qualified and who represented the

Royal Colleges, the Universities and the Privy Council. This Act was intended in part to enable 'persons requiring medical aid [to be] . . . enabled to distinguish qualified from unqualified practitioners'. In order to achieve this a register was created.

Subsequent Medical Acts — the most recent being the Medical Act 1983 which consolidates the previous Acts — have expanded the role and thus the workload of the GMC. Its activities are limited to carrying out powers and duties conferred by statute. As such its actions may be subject to public law challenge by the route of judicial review. The GMC summarises its current role by stating that:

. . . the general duty of the Council is to protect the public and to uphold the reputation of the profession. The Council does this by keeping and publishing the Register of qualified doctors, by fixing the standard of education and experience required for entry to the Register and by promoting high standards of medical education, by giving advice to doctors on standards of professional conduct and on medical ethics, and by taking action against registered doctors if it appears that they have become unfit to practise and to continue to exercise the privileges of registration.

Despite much dispute an Independent Committee of Inquiry reported in 1975,[b] recommending the continuation of 'self-regulation' by the profession — that is, that the majority of GMC members be elected by those medical practitioners whose names appear on the Medical Register. The majority of the GMC's income is derived from registration of new members and from the annual retention fees of existing members.

Structure of GMC

The GMC has 102 members. 54 are elected, 35 appointed and 13 are nominated. The Medical Act 1978 established that the number of elected members should exceed the number of nominated or appointed members. Elected members are medically qualified and elections take place every 5 years. In 1994 25% of newly elected doctors were less than 45 years of age, 11 of 54 were overseas qualified and 13 were female.[c]

Appointed members are appointed by bodies which grant registrable qualifications (e.g. Royal Colleges and Universities), and each is medically qualified.

Nominated members are lay members (defined as those who have no medical qualifications) and are nominated by the Queen on the advice of the Privy Council, and like appointed members serve for up to 5 years. Prior to April 1994 two of the nominated members were medically qualified (two of the four Chief Medical Officers), but in order to provide extra places for lay members this no longer happens. The GMC is currently consulting on changes to the structure, which include proposals to increase the number of lay members to about 25% of the total, partially in response to society's perceived desire for '. . . growing lay involvement in the regulation of the professions',[d] and also because of the practical implications of the introduction of professional performance procedures (see below).

Functions of the GMC

The Register

The registration system allows all qualified medical practitioners to be identified for legal and official purposes. The Register of Medical Practitioners allows the public to identify properly qualified medical practitioners and is the means by which the GMC is enabled to carry out its professional conduct and educational roles. The Register shows a doctor's full name, sex, primary qualifications, and additional higher qualifications. UK qualified doctors are provisionally registered for the first year after qualifying and after satisfactory completion of the 'pre-registration' year, are granted full registration.

The Register of Medical Practitioners is divided into four separate lists. The Principal List contains details of doctors, the majority of whom are resident in the UK. The Overseas List includes all those living outside the UK and the European Union and thus exempted from a retention fee. The Visiting Overseas Doctors List is small and contains the names of overseas qualified doctors who have been granted temporary full registration as they are providing specialist medical services. The Visiting European Union Practitioners List contains the names of a small number of doctors visiting the UK to provide specialist medical services.

Certain other doctors qualified outside the UK and European Union may be eligible for provisional or limited registration. Eligibility for full, limited, or provisional registration is determined partly by the Medical Act 1983 and also by regulations and decisions of the GMC. Factors that can be taken into account include the recognition of degrees granted by overseas examining bodies, professional skills and knowledge of the English language.

Education

The Medical Act 1983 consolidated the powers of the Medical Act 1978 endowing the Education Committee of the Council with responsibility for 'determining the knowledge and skill to be required for the granting of registrable medical qualifications in the United Kingdom and the standard of proficiency to be required from candidates at qualifying examinations for such qualifications'.[e]

The Council can therefore make representations to the Privy Council to consider either conferring or withdrawing approval as to the standard of an institution's qualifications in terms of suitability for registration. The Education Committee is empowered to seek information (on an annual basis) on curricula and examinations from all Examining Bodies and medical schools.

The Education Committee can review hospitals, patterns of experience, or combinations of posts for doctors in their pre-registration year, and may notify the University which has approved the post(s) if they are considered unsuitable. The University is obliged to take into account that opinion.

A number of additional postgraduate higher degrees or diplomas granted in the United Kingdom are now recognised for registration. These include masters degrees in surgery, doctorates in medicine and membership of the Royal Colleges of Physicians, Pathologists, Psychiatrists and General Practitioners, and fellowship of the Royal Colleges of Surgeons and Anaesthetists. For the purposes of registration a completion certificate by the appropriate training body of higher specialist training is also recognised.

The Education Committee has an additional function of 'promoting high standards of medical education and co-ordinating all stages of medical education'. Thus the Committee should ensure the unity of all stages of training — from undergraduate level through to continuing medical education after the specialist training has been completed.

Under a European Community Directive mutual recognition of certain primary and specialist[f] medical qualifications was outlined, which also permitted unrestricted movement of doctors between member countries. These directives were given effect by the Medical Qualification (EEC Recognition) Order 1977, SI 1977/827, and required the GMC to grant full registration to nationals of member countries with primary medical qualifications.

The issue of 'specialist training' has been an area of concern, whereby 'accreditation' in the UK (the means by which recognition of training within the UK to a specialist level has been completed) in effect requires a longer period of training than that required in other member states. A legal challenge about the requirements for 'specialist' training raised a number of interesting legalistic problems but no ruling was made on the apparent fact that the GMC had contravened EC law by acknowledging that there was a difference in standards.[1]

In January 1996, under the European Specialist Medical Qualifications Order 1995, the GMC was required to establish and publish a Specialist Register, inclusion in which will be determined by a new Specialist Training Authority.

Conduct procedures

The Medical Act 1983 created three Committees which are directly involved in undertaking the GMC's responsibilities in relation to professional conduct and fitness to practise. These are the Preliminary Proceedings Committee (PPC), the Professional Conduct Committee (PCC) and the Health Committee.

Complaints are examined in the first instance by 'preliminary screeners' of which three are medically qualified and two are lay. Screeners have a number of functions. One key function, often misunderstood, is to decide whether the complaint is one that lies within the GMC's jurisdiction. All complaints are screened. If the complaint lies beyond the GMC's statutory function (as agreed by both a medical and lay screener), the complainant is contacted and where appropriate advised about the correct route for the particular complaint (see Ch. 3).

Once it has been decided that the complaint falls within the GMC's remit, the evidence is assessed (in some cases after further inquiries or consultation with other screeners, or Council members) to determine whether the doctor may have committed serious professional misconduct. If the evidence suggests that this may be the case, the complaint is referred to the PPC.

If the screener is of the opinion that there is not enough evidence to support an allegation of serious professional misconduct, but there are still grounds for concern, then the doctor against whom the complaint is made is requested to make comments on the allegation. Dependent on the doctor's comments, again a lay and medical screener in agreement may conclude the complaint by

---

1 R v *Joint Committee on Higher Medical Training and Specialist Advisory Committee on Rheumatology, ex parte Goldstein* [1992] BMLR (CA) 11 10–20

issuing advice to the doctor on future conduct. Thus formal disciplinary proceedings may be avoided.

What constitutes serious professional misconduct? Prior to the Medical Act 1969 the phrase 'infamous conduct in a professional respect' was used. Two judgments are quoted when attempting to define this phrase and are used now to define serious professional misconduct. Lord Justice Lopes in *Allinson*[2] stated, '. . . if it is shown that a medical man, in the pursuit of his profession, has done something with regard to it which would be reasonably regarded as disgraceful or dishonourable by his professional brethren of good repute and competency'. This was in relation to Dr Allinson having advertised to the public telling them to have nothing to do with other practitioners. Subsequently in 1930 Lord Justice Scrutton stated, '. . . infamous conduct . . . means no more than serious misconduct according to the rules, written or unwritten, governing the profession.'[3]

The PPC considers cases that have been referred by the preliminary screeners and also criminal cases where doctors have been convicted of an offence. The PPC has 12 members (10 medical and two lay). The PPC considers the evidence of the complainant and the doctor (who will have been invited to submit a written explanation of events). The PPC may decide to take one of a number of courses of action including: referring the case to the PCC; taking no further action; sending a letter of advice on future conduct to the doctor; or referring the doctor to the Health Committee for further investigation. In certain cases that it deems appropriate the PPC can suspend a doctor's registration, or impose conditions on practice for an interim period of up to 2 months. The doctor is allowed to challenge such an order, and may be legally represented.

Box 2.1 gives examples of professional conduct and personal behaviour which can or could give rise to disciplinary proceedings.[g] These have been expanded by the recent publication of the booklet *Good Medical Practice*,[h] which is part of the GMC's Standards Committee's 3-part revision of the guidance to doctors on standards of conduct. *Good Medical Practice* expands on a more concise booklet — *The Duties of a Doctor*.[i] These duties are summarised in Box 2.2. The third booklet — *Confidentiality* — details the principles of confidentiality expected to be observed by practitioners.[j]

2 *Allinson* v *General Council of Medical Education & Registration* [1894] 1 QB 750
3 *R* v *General Council of Medical Education & Registration of the United Kingdom* [1930] 1 KB 562

Box 2.1 Potential reasons for disciplinary proceedings (adapted with permission from Professional Conduct and Fitness to Practise, GMC, 1993)

- Neglect or disregard by doctors of their professional responsibilities to patients for their care and treatment: e.g. failing to visit a patient; failing to provide treatment; failing to arrange treatment; improperly delegating work to a person who is not a registered medical practitioner

- Abuse of professional privileges conferred by law or custom or abuse of professional skills: e.g. prescribing or supplying drugs of dependence inappropriately; issuing medical certificates inappropriately; inappropriate termination of pregnancy; disclosure of confidential information; entering into emotional or sexual relationships with a patient

- Personal behaviour — conduct derogatory to the reputation of the profession: e.g. drunkenness/misuse of alcohol; treating patients under the influence of drugs or alcohol; criminal deception; fraud; forgery; charging fees to National Health Service patients; prescribing/dispensing drugs or appliances in which the doctor has a financial interest; indecent or violent behaviour

- Advertising doctors' services: e.g. misleading information; disparaging other practitioners; exerting pressure on individuals to become patients

- Comment on professional colleagues: e.g. gratuitous comment attempting to undermine trust in a colleague's skills

---

The PCC has 32 members (26 medical, six lay). Cases are heard by 11 members, generally in public. The PCC's role is to protect the public and uphold the reputation of the medical profession. As with criminal justice proceedings in a court of law, the cases are adversarial. The proceedings are governed by rules made by the GMC following consultation with professional and patient bodies. Appeals go to the Privy Council. If the proceedings come about as a result of

---

Box 2.2 Duties of a doctor. Reproduced by permission from General Medical Council 1995 The duties of a doctor. GMC, London

As a doctor you must:

- make the care of your patient your first concern;
- treat every patient with courtesy and consideration;
- respect patients' dignity and privacy;
- listen to patients and respect their views;
- give patients information in a way they can understand;
- respect the right of patients to be fully involved in decisions about their care;
- keep your professional knowledge and skills up to date;
- recognise the limits of your professional competence;
- be honest and worthy of trust;
- respect and protect confidential information;
- make sure that your personal beliefs do not prejudice your patient's care;
- act quickly to protect patients from risk if you have good reason to believe that you or a colleague may be unfit to practise;
- avoid abuse of your position as a doctor;
- work with colleagues in the ways that best serve patients' interests.

---

criminal proceedings in which the doctor admitted the offence or was found guilty then the PCC assesses the evidence to determine the gravity of the proceedings, and whether there were mitigating factors. If the proceedings come about as a result of a complaint about conduct, the PCC decides on the facts before it whether or not the doctor was guilty of serious professional misconduct. The standard of proof is that of the criminal court — the case must be proved 'beyond reasonable doubt'. If during the course of the proceeding it becomes evident that the doctor's fitness to practise is possibly impaired due to physical or mental health reasons, the case may be referred to the Health Committee. If the Health Committee finds that this is the case, the PCC takes no further action.

If the PCC finds a doctor guilty of serious professional misconduct (or finds that a doctor has been convicted of a criminal offence) a number of outcomes are possible. The case may be concluded or the PCC may postpone its determination. In the latter case the doctor may be expected to provide references at the resumed hearing from colleagues concerning his conduct since the previous hearing. If these are satisfactory the case may be concluded. The PCC may decide that the doctor's registration is conditional on compliance (for no more than 3 years) with specific requirements imposed by the PCC (e.g. not prescribing controlled drugs; not undertaking private practice; undergoing a period of retraining in a particular skill). If the doctor complies satisfactorily, the conditional registration may be lifted. If not, suspension or erasure from the Register may be directed. The PCC may direct that suspension (preventing a doctor from practising) takes place immediately for a period, but the case can be reconsidered before the end of the suspension period — although either erasure or conditional registration can still be imposed. The PCC can direct that the doctor's name is erased from the Medical Register. A doctor may apply to be restored to the Register, 10 months after the original order. If that application is unsuccessful a further 10-month period must elapse. Notice of appeal against any of these sanctions must be made, within 28 days of the order, to the Judicial Committee of the Privy Council. It is worth noting that the opinion has been expressed that an 'appellate tribunal should be slow to interfere with a professional body's exercise of discretion as to sentence.'[4] Tables 2.1 and 2.2 summarise the data from 1994 concerning Conduct Procedures and outcomes.

Physical or mental health impairment

The GMC has laid down procedures for rehabilitation of doctors whose fitness to practise is seriously impaired by illness. These procedures are statute-based[k,l]. They are intended to protect patients from doctors whose fitness to practise is impaired by ill-health, to provide monitoring and care with a goal of returning them to unrestricted practice, and to maintain the confidentiality that any ill individual may be owed.

A variety of sources may bring the doctor's health to the notice of the GMC. Frequently the source is concerned colleagues, but other agencies such as hospitals, police, courts or patients may

---

4 Lord Parker in: *Marten v Disciplinary Committee of the Royal College of Veterinary Surgeons* [1966] 1 QB 1; [1965] 1 All ER 949

Table 2.1 Cases considered by the Preliminary Proceedings Committee in 1994 (from GMC Annual Report 1994)

Nature of Case	Source		Totals	Outcome					
	Conviction	Alleged serious professional misconduct		Adjourned to a meeting in 1995	No action	Letter of advice or admonition	Adjourned sine die (health procedures)	Referred to Health Committee	PCC
Treatment by NHS GPs	0	35	35	2	0	14	1	0	18
Indecency, etc	7	15	22	0	2	5	1	0	14
Abuse of alcohol/drugs	17	3	20	0	0	11	9	0	0
Breach of professional confidence	0	11	11	0	2	9	0	0	0
Dishonesty/fraud/deception	11	0	11	1	0	1	2	0	7
Improper relationships	0	10	10	1	1	2	1	0	5
Irresponsible prescribing	0	9	9	0	0	1	0	1	7
False or improper certification	0	8	8	0	0	2	0	0	6
Advertising	0	8	8	0	0	8	0	0	2
Hospital treatment under NHS	0	7	7	0	0	3	2	0	2
False claims to qualifications or experience	0	7	7	0	0	1	0	0	6
Violent/abusive behaviour	4	3	7	0	1	4	2	0	0
Falsifying medical records or reports	0	5	5	0	0	1	1	0	3
Miscellaneous motoring convictions	5	0	5	1	0	4	0	0	0
Misconduct in drug trial	0	4	4	0	0	1	0	0	3
Rudeness	0	3	3	0	1	0	2	0	0
Failure to provide specimen of breath	3	0	3	1	0	2	0	0	0
Improperly charging for NHS services	0	3	3	0	0	2	0	0	3
Undue influence over patients	0	2	2	0	0	2	0	0	0
Illegal supply of drugs/seeking to obtain drugs by deception	1	1	2	0	0	0	0	0	2
Manslaughter	2	0	2	0	0	0	0	0	2
Impeding due inquiry	0	2	2	0	0	1	0	0	1
Seeking to obtain loans from patients	0	1	1	0	0	0	0	0	1
Failure to report misconduct by colleague	0	1	1	0	0	0	0	0	1
Pretending to be a registered medical practitioner	0	1	1	0	0	1	0	0	0
Failure to provide medical reports	0	1	1	0	0	1	0	0	0
Inadequate practice arrangements	0	1	1	0	0	0	0	0	1
Disparagement	0	1	1	0	0	0	1	0	0
Non-NHS treatment	0	1	1	0	0	0	0	0	0
Failure to obtain consent to treatment	0	1	1	0	1	0	0	0	0
Failure to comply with provisions of Mental Health Act	0	1	1	0	1	0	0	0	0
Totals	**50**	**145**	**195**	**6**	**9**	**74**	**22**	**1**	**83**

Table 2.2 Work of the Professional Conduct Committee in 1994 (from GMC Annual Report 1994)

Nature of Case	Source Convictions	Alleged serious professional misconduct	Totals	Outcome Not guilty of SPM	Admonished and/or case concluded	Conditional registration	Suspension	Erasure	Erasure with immediate suspension
Disregard of professional responsibilities to patients	0	26	26	3	8(3R)	8(1R)	5(1R)	2(1R)	0
Indecency, etc	4	9	13	2	0	0	2	4	5
Financial dishonesty/theft	6	4	10	1	4(1R)	2	0	3	0
Irresponsible prescribing	0	7	7	0	1(1R)	2	0	1	3
False claims to qualifications or experience	0	6	6	1	1	0	1	2	1
Improper emotional/sexual relationship with patients	0	6	6	2	0	1	0	3	0
Fraudulent returns in clinical drugs trial	0	3	3	0	0	1	1	1	0
False certification	0	3	3	0	1	0	0	1	1
Charging for NHS services	0	2	2	0	1	0	0	0	0
Improper alteration of medical records	1	0	1	0	0	0	0	1	0
Using instruments to procure miscarriages	0	1	1	0	0	0	0	1	0
Failure to obtain consent to treatment	0	1	1	0	1	0	0	0	0
Failure to report misconduct of colleague	0	1	1	0	0	0	0	0	0
Breach of professional confidence	0	1	1	1	0	0	1	0	0
Manslaughter	1	0	1	0	0	0	1	0	0
Inadequate practice arrangements	0	1	1	0	0	1	0	0	0
Undue influence on patients to lend money	0	1	1	0	0	0	0	1	0
Totals	**12**	**72**	**84**	**10**	**19**	**15**	**10**	**19**	**11**

1 Figures shown in brackets and marked (1R, 2R, etc) denote the number of cases included in total which were resumed from an earlier hearing in 1994 or a previous year

2 Where a doctor appeared before the Committee to face charges in relation to more than one matter (e.g. disregard of professional responsibilities and dishonesty), this is shown above as two or more separate cases

instigate action. The case is assessed by a screener who may conclude that there is a health problem and will invite the doctor to be examined by two nominated medical examiners. They give an opinion on whether the doctor is fit to practise without restriction, and may make recommendations, often including medical care and treatment, supervision or limitations on practice. If the doctor accepts the recommendations, the doctor supervising treatment will make reports to the screener. If the health problem improves then the limitations on practice may be removed until, ideally, fitness to practise without supervision is allowed.

If the doctor fails to cooperate, fails to follow the recommendations on treatment and limitations on practice, or ill-health becomes apparent during either PPC or PCC proceedings, the case is referred to the Health Committee. Alcohol and drug misuse and mental health problems are the most common causes of referral to the Health Committee.[m] The Committee has 12 members (11 medical, one lay) and is advised by specialist medical assessors. Although this Committee's proceedings (which are held in private) are not adversarial, the doctor may be legally represented, and witnesses may be called. If the Committee decides that the doctor's fitness to practise is seriously impaired, it can impose conditional registration (e.g. to accept medical treatment) for up to three years, or suspend registration for up to a year. The Health Committee cannot erase from the Register. Each case is reconsidered before the end of conditional or suspended registration. Appeals may be made to the Judicial Committee of the Privy Council.

Poor performance

The fact that there has been no conduct 'offence' less than serious professional misconduct has been a concern of many. The lack of sanctions against doctors whose work whilst poor or inadequate has not been sufficient to warrant a consideration of serious professional misconduct is intended to be corrected in a new Bill which had its first reading in the House of Commons in March 1995. The Medical (Professional Performance) Act passed on November 8 1995 amends the Medical Act 1983 and gives the GMC new jurisdiction over the professional competence of doctors. In particular the Act introduces the concept of 'seriously deficient standard of professional performance'. The term is not defined. In summary, complaints about a doctor whose standard of professional performance is considered to be seriously deficient will be screened by a medical member of the GMC. If assessment is recommended but refused the doctor will be referred to the new Assessment Referral Committee (ARC). This will have the power to order assessment, and any deficiencies thus identified will be remedied by retraining and reassessment. The Committee on Professional Performance (CPP) will be created to deal with those cases that have not been satisfactorily concluded or where the doctor has refused assessment, and will have the power to impose conditions or suspend registration. Detailed rules on this complex procedure have yet to be finalized, and following pilot tests in 1996 the procedures are expected to be underway in 1997.

UNITED KINGDOM CENTRAL COUNCIL (UKCC)

The United Kingdom Central Council (UKCC) was formed by the Nurses', Midwives', and Health Visitors' Act of 1979 as the regulating body of these professions. It is responsible by law for establishing and improving standards of training, conduct and practice, and as such keeps a register of all practitioners. The Council has sole power for conferring registration and for removing a practitioner from the register on grounds of misconduct or unfitness to practise.

The Council is made up of 40 elected members (including seven nurses, two midwives and one health visitor from each country) and 20 members appointed by the Secretary of State for Health.

All members of the nursing profession are required to practise within the Code of Professional Conduct issued and regularly updated by the Council.[n] Recommendations for change and improvement of the Code are welcomed by the Council from any member of the nursing professions.

Professional conduct

The Nurses, Midwives, and Health Visitors Act 1992 conferred additional responsibilities on the Council in respect of professional conduct affairs. The Council is required to make Statutory Rules which control the conditions and means by which a person's name may be removed from the register. These rules require the setting up of Committees of members to consider allegations of misconduct or unfitness to practise against registered practitioners.

A Preliminary Proceedings Committee determines whether cases of alleged misconduct should be dismissed or referred for a hearing by the Professional Conduct Committee. Cases concerning fitness to practise are first dealt with by a Professional Screenings Meeting who will either dismiss the case or forward it for hearing by the Health Committee. Both the Professional Conduct and the Health Committees have powers of suspension or removal from the register. Referral between Committees for misconduct and fitness to practise can be made.

Complaints alleging misconduct or unfitness to practise can be made by anyone and should be sent in writing to the Council.⁰

Misconduct

In the case of misconduct an officer of the Council will then assemble evidence. The accused practitioner will be asked for a written statement, explanation or comment. Criminal conviction will occasionally form the basis on which the case proceeds. The practitioner will not normally be called in person unless interim suspension is being considered. The Committees have two main tasks when dealing with allegations of misconduct; to decide whether facts alleged against the practitioner are proved 'beyond reasonable doubt', and to decide whether the proved facts constitute misconduct. Professional Conduct Committees have legal assessors in attendance, and the accused practitioner may be represented. The hearing is held in public. Examples of offences which may lead to removal from the register include: concealing untoward incidents, falsifying records, failure to protect or promote interests of patients and physical or verbal abuse of a patient.

Fitness

Along with the written allegation, brief details of the illness and identity of the practitioner should be sent to the Council. The Council's solicitor then draws up a statutory declaration for the accuser to sign. Only upon receipt of this can the investigation legally proceed. The Panel of Screeners then decide from the documentary evidence which specialist medical examiners to refer the practitioner to. From their findings the Panel will judge whether to refer the case to the Health Committee, the Preliminary Proceedings Committee, or the Professional Conduct Committee (if that is where the referral came from originally) or whether the case should be closed. The medical findings are available to the practitioner, and they may choose to commission additional reports from a practitioner of their own choice. The Committees' main task is to judge whether the practitioner's fitness is impaired so as to be a 'likely danger to the vulnerable public'. Because of their nature, Health Committee hearings are private. The most frequent conditions which have led to removal from the register are alcohol and other drug dependence, and various mental illnesses.

SUMMARY

It is clear that the climate of opinion in today's society recognises that the public has concerns about how professions regulate themselves. The perception that self-regulation might work against the interests of the consumer was in the past perhaps well founded. This appears less so now, and it is of note that many bodies are attempting to ensure that the best possible service is provided by practitioners. The Council of the College of Speech and Language Therapists, for example, has published a substantial book of professional guidelines, directed not merely to the profession but to those who use its services.[p] This perhaps is a model on which guidelines from other professions could be based.

It is the use of such information, enabling the public to understand what the particular profession expects of its own practitioners, that might enable inappropriate complaints to be reduced. More importantly it may identify practitioners who fail to come up to their own peers' standards, and thus action to remedy the situation can be instigated.

REFERENCES

a   General Medical Council 1991 Constitution and functions. General Medical Council, London
b   Report of the Committee of Inquiry into the regulation of the medical profession, Cmnd 6018 (Merrison Report) 1975. HMSO, London
c   GMC Election 1994. The GMC News Review 1994: 5: 1. General Medical Council, London
d   General Medical Council 1994 The composition of the General Medical Council: proposals for change. A consultation paper. General Medical Council, London
e   General Medical Council 1991 Constitution and functions. General Medical Council, London
f   EC Directive No. 75/363 (the Second Medical Directive) of the Council of European Communities

g General Medical Council 1993 Professional conduct and discipline: fitness to practise. General Medical Council, London
h General Medical Council 1995 Good medical practice. General Medical Council, London
i General Medical Council 1995 The duties of a doctor. General Medical Council, London
j General Medical Council 1995 Confidentiality. General Medical Council, London
k Medical Act 1983, Part V and Schedule 4
l Health Committee (Procedure) Rules 1987. SI1987 No. 2174. HMSO, London
m Allibone A 1993 The work of the Health Committee (GMC Annual Report). General Medical Council, London
n United Kingdom Central Council 1992 Code of professional conduct for the nurse, midwife and health visitor, 3rd edn. United Kingdom Central Council, London
o United Kingdom Central Council 1993 Complaints about professional conduct. United Kingdom Central Council, London
p College of Speech and Language Therapists 1991 Communicating quality: professional standards for speech and language therapists. College of Speech and Language Therapists, London

3. Complaints in the National Health Service

Simon Payne

INTRODUCTION

The right to complain is one of the fundamental features of a civilised society and is a cornerstone of democracy. This chapter outlines complaint procedures related to healthcare in the UK. In parallel with other changes in administrative law leading to greater openness in practice within the National Health Service in recent years, a number of developments have occurred in relation to NHS complaints which provide for a stronger framework for public rights. Alongside the Access to Medical Reports Act 1989 and the Access to Health Records Act 1990, which effectively provide for the patient the right to gain access to their case records and reports written about them (with certain minor limitations) virtually on demand, the Patient's Charter[a] provides for patients using NHS services the right to obtain from the hospital a prompt written reply within time limits of approximately 1 month for any complaint that the patient may have regarding NHS services used. The complaint may be made in writing or verbally and in the latter case the expectation is that the hospital administration will make provision for a verbal complaint to be transcribed and investigated as fully as if it had been received in the form of a letter.

A further development for the NHS is the implementation of the Wilson Report,[b] provisions of which are scheduled to be fully complied with for all clinical matters by 1 April 1996.

Reasons behind a complaint in the NHS

In its broadest perspective, a complaint involving an issue arising out of NHS practice is always driven by dissatisfaction. This in turn occurs because the recipient of the service believes that something has gone wrong with their treatment.

The relationship between the healthcare professionals in providing services and the general public who are the recipients as patients is not an equal one. The power balance is stacked in the favour of the providers, whose knowledge and elevation places them in a position of extreme strength over the patient, who may be completely ignorant of the medical implications of their condition and may find their vulnerability further undermined by the incapacitating nature of the condition. It is because of this imbalance that the various types of complaints procedure which exist may sometimes appear to favour the complainant.

Framework of complaints

Complaints within the NHS may take one of the following forms:

- Hospital complaint
- General practitioner (GP) complaint
- Disciplinary action
- Civil litigation
- Criminal prosecution.

The above procedures may be invoked singularly or in combination depending on the nature of the matter about which the complaint has arisen.

Broadly speaking, hospital complaints and GP complaints may arise either from administrative issues or perceived clinical failures. Matters of professional conduct may also be included in hospital and GP complaints, although this is uncommon.

Internal disciplinary action may be undertaken against a member of staff following a hospital complaint, and if the issues concerned are considered to be of a sufficiently serious nature the matter may be reported to a professional body governing the healthcare professional involved (see Ch. 2).

Criminal proceedings may be taken following a complaint to the police by a patient that a criminal act has taken place in the course of a professional consultation. Such events are rare and would almost invariably involve allegations of indecent assault on a female patient by a male doctor. More recently two sinister developments have occurred in criminal proceedings affecting the medical profession. Recent well-publicised cases[1, 2] have demonstrated

---

1 R v Adomako [1994] 1956 (HL), P
2 R v Cox [1992] 1238, Crown Ct.

the increased willingness of the criminal prosecution system to bring criminal proceedings against medical practitioners where disastrous outcomes of treatment (usually involving death of the patient) occur, the like of which would hitherto have been considered to be civil matters. An important difference between the civil and criminal codes is highlighted by this development, namely that in civil litigation the aim is to compensate loss suffered by the plaintiff, whereas criminal proceedings seek primarily to punish the defendant for wrongdoing. In both codes the burden of proof rests with the individual or agency prosecuting the crime or tort. However, in criminal matters the standard of proof is significantly higher; that is to say, the convicting jury are required to be 'satisfied so they are sure' ('beyond reasonable doubt') as opposed to the 'balance of probabilities test' which is applied by the judge who decides a civil action.

A further area of liability of which doctors should be aware relates to the sequelae of a criminal conviction of any kind. It is a standing requirement of the criminal courts that any conviction brought against a medical practitioner registered with the General Medical Council (GMC), whether or not this has arisen through the practice of medicine, must be reported to the GMC, who will consider the facts and will decide whether any additional disciplinary action against the individual concerned should be taken.

Hospital complaints

These may be received in verbal or written form.[c] When receiving a verbal complaint the hospital is expected to transcribe it into a written form and to deal with it accordingly.

Hospital complaints are divided into two categories — clinical and non-clinical.

Non-clinical complaints

For non-clinical complaints there is no question of failure of clinical judgment but the complainant perceives a failure in some administrative part of the system which has led to inconvenience, suffering or loss.

The hospital should have a designated complaints officer who supervises an investigation into the details of the complaint, and this should lead to a written reply to the complainant signed by the Chief Executive and sent promptly following receipt of the original complaint. Under normal circumstances this letter is expected to be sent within 30 days.[d]

The above process satisfies most complainants, but for those who remain dissatisfied following a letter of explanation from the Chief Executive an appeals procedure exists. This involves the Health Service Ombudsman and a decision must be made by the hospital as to whether the matter in hand is one which ought properly be dealt by the Ombudsman. The 'end of the road' will be reached either if the hospital decides that the matter in hand is not one which ought properly be dealt by the Ombudsman or if the Ombudsman upholds the hospital's position on the complaint in question.

Clinical complaints

Perceived failure in clinical matters may be dealt with either in the clinical complaints procedure or through the civil courts.

To be dealt with in the civil courts the matter must satisfy the requirements of negligence (see Ch. 13), that is to say that there has been a breach of a duty of care resulting in damage to the patient and that the damage which has occurred is a direct result of the breach of duty. The standards of care applied in a case considered in negligence are those laid down in Bolam.[3] That is to say the practitioner concerned is expected to have displayed the level of skill of the average practitioner trained in the particular clinical speciality concerned. The purpose of such an action in negligence is to seek financial compensation for the loss which has occurred. It follows, therefore, that for an action in negligence to be pursued the patient must have suffered some form of loss as a direct result of an act or omission of a member of the healthcare team who has been involved in providing diagnosis or treatment. A further practical prerequisite for a case in negligence being brought is that the patient/plaintiff must be in a position to support the legal costs of the claim that is being made. In the event that the plaintiff wins his case it is usual that his costs will be met by the defendant, which in such a case is the hospital concerned. On the other hand if the case does not succeed then the plaintiff will be liable for their costs and disbursements, which may be very considerable indeed especially if the case proceeds to trial. It follows, therefore, that cases which may have some merit in negligence are sometimes not

3 Bolam v Friern Hospital Management Committee [1957] 1 WLR 582

brought because the plaintiff is neither wealthy enough to afford the costs nor poor enough to qualify for legal aid.

The existing arrangements for dealing with clinical complaints not involving litigation include a three stage procedure.[e]

Stage I involves a discussion between the consultant in charge of the case and the complainant. Clinical facts of the case are established as far as is possible and the consultant concerned should take a view regarding the adequacy of the clinical performance of the individuals involved and should explain the position as sympathetically as possible to the complainant. This procedure may satisfy the complainant in a proportion of cases. However, if the complainant remains dissatisfied then the matter proceeds to Stage II.

Stage II — Clinical complaints: here the consultant will report the proceedings of Stage I to the hospital administrators and may also involve the Regional Director of Public Health. Following discussions the complainant may be further interviewed and/or offered a written explanation of the situation. Should the complainant remain dissatisfied at this stage it is then a matter for the Regional Director of Public Health to decide whether or not an independent professional review is appropriate.

Stage III — Clinical complaints: this procedure involves inviting consultants in the relevant speciality from outside the local area to review and assess the details of the case and complaint. The assessors report to the Regional Director of Public Health who in turn briefs the Chief Executive of the hospital concerned. Armed with this independent review and opinion on the performance of the clinical staff concerned, the Chief Executive will write a further letter to the complainant. This completes the hospital complaints procedure for clinical matters. Should the patient at this stage continue to be dissatisfied, a decision is then made as to whether the appeals procedure should be enacted. This involves a referral of the papers to the Health Service Ombudsman who will further assess and adjudicate on the case. It is possible that the patient remains dissatisfied even after this stage, but should this occur, no further procedures are available and the matter has once again reached the 'end of the road'. A dissatisfied complainant in this position may only seek redress in the civil courts if they wish to take the matter further.

The recommendations of the Wilson Report[b] seek to modify the above procedures to improve the accessibility, simplicity, speed and responsiveness of the way in which complaints are dealt with.

In essence, the proposed new complaints procedure for both hospital complaints and GP complaints is envisaged as conforming to a two-stage process. The purpose of Stage I under the new Wilson proposals involves an attempt to engineer a more informal and internal procedure including a dialogue between the complainant and front-line clinical staff and/or managers, prompt investigation of the problems and an attempt at conciliation with written response from senior partners (general practice), complaints officers and/or FHSA/Trust Chief Executives.

In the event that Stage I fails, i.e. that the complainant remains dissatisfied, a screening procedure is envisaged in which the performance of Stage I of the complaint is reviewed and a decision is made as to whether the matter could still be undertaken under Stage I parameters.

A decision is also made by the screener as to whether the matter may be more appropriately dealt with under disciplinary procedures.

The substantive part of a Stage II procedure under the new Wilson proposals involves the independent review of issues raised in the complaint by a panel. It is recommended that the panel should be normally composed of three members but that if the complaint raises issues of professional judgment or requires particular specialist knowledge, two additional members may be appointed. These two members should be included from the relevant speciality and should act as independent assessors of the clinical details in a similar way to the independent professional review under the old Stage III clinical complaints procedure (as currently existing).[f]

Under Wilson the panel is empowered to investigate the complaint and make recommendations, reporting both to the complainant and the relevant Chief Executive(s). The Chief Executive is then expected to undertake necessary management action and if appropriate to report the matter to the relevant professional organisation. It is expected that the new procedure will complete its investigation and report within 5 weeks from the date of complaint.

General practice complaints

The existing GP complaints procedure which is also intended to be modified under Wilson recommendations differs significantly from NHS hospital complaints processes, in that the GP complaints process is couched in terms of breach of contract. General practitioners differ from hospital practitioners in that the former are employed under a contract for services while the latter are employed under a contract of service. GPs are therefore independent contractors and thus not as easily subject to disciplinary controls as their hospital counterparts.

A complaint made to the Family Health Service Authority (FHSA) is dealt with as a potential breach of contract. Under their contract for services, GPs undertake to provide 'all necessary medical services' for the patients on their list. Failure to do so, if upheld in the GP complaints procedure, leads to a withholding of payment in respect of the services contracted. In such circumstances, therefore, the GP is in effect financially penalised for a failure in the service which may be of an administrative nature, a disciplinary nature or even in clinical standards. The rules regarding multiple jeopardy apply to GPs in the sense that a complaint which is upheld and leads to a withholding of remuneration may also be brought to the attention of the practitioners' disciplinary body (GMC), may be raised as an issue in the civil courts in negligence, and may on rare occasions also attract criminal prosecution.

The mechanism of the GP complaints procedure is as follows.[g]

Following a complaint to the FHSA, a decision is made as to whether the matter may be dealt with informally or following the formal complaints procedure. The informal conciliation approach is usually followed when the complaints are estimated by the preliminary screening process as not amounting to a possible breach of terms of service. Even where a possible breach of terms of service is felt to apply by the preliminary screening process, it is possible for the complaint to be dealt with informally, provided the FHSA agrees. In the event that the complainant does not wish to follow this route, or following informal conciliation the complainant remains dissatisfied and the matter is felt to amount to a possible breach of terms of service, then these cases are referred to a Service Committee for consideration.

The Service Committee is composed of a lay Chair but contains also both lay and professional members from the Medical, Dental, Pharmaceutical and Ophthalmic professions. The Committee takes both written and oral evidence, and both complainant (patient) and defendant (doctor) may be accompanied by a 'friend' who may obtain assistance in representing their case or defence provided that this is not produced by a 'paid advocate'. An attempt is, therefore, made to avoid a quasi-judicial forum by the avoidance, as far as is possible, of lawyers.

The decision of the Service Committee is referred for confirmation to the FHSA, and if this is adverse to the GP a right of appeal exists to the Secretary of State for Health. Should the complainant remain dissatisfied after the decision of the Service Committee confirmed by the FHSA, appeal is also possible to the Secretary of State for Health. On considering the details of the matter the Secretary of State is empowered either to increase or reduce the withholding of remuneration that has been recommended by the FHSA.

Summary

Complaints of various kinds are the mechanism by which the users of the Health Service make known to the organisation of that service their dissatisfaction with perceived failures. Although frequently the underlying problem is a failure of communication, there are occasions when true deficiencies are uncovered. The expectation of the modern and reformed Health Service in the United Kingdom is for the issues raised to be taken seriously in a timely and effective manner. The positive approach which is promoted is primarily designed to rectify deficiencies and educate those whose acts or omissions may have led to the problem. The complaints procedure should acknowledge the problem that has been raised by the complainant, provide an apology where appropriate (although this is not synonymous with admission of liability), should provide an explanation of the events which have been experienced by the patient, and should notify the complainant both of the final conclusions of the investigation precipitated by the complaint and any positive action or specific measures which have been undertaken as a result of the matters drawn to the attention of the authority in the course of the complaint.

REFERENCES

a   Citizen's Charter Complaints Taskforce 1990 Effective complaints systems: principles and checklist. Citizen's Charter Unit, London
b   Wilson A 1994 Report of a review committee on NHS complaints procedures (The Wilson Report). Department of Health, London
c   Ibid p.38
d   Ibid p.38
e   Department of Health Circular HC(88)37. Department of Health, London
f   Ibid
g   General Medical Council 1990 Working for patients. HMSO, London

4. Consent to medical treatment

Anthony Barton

INTRODUCTION

Consent to medical treatment is a large subject and concerns such diverse matters as the relationships between ethics and law, law and medicine, the lay person and the professional, the individual and the state and the parent and the child. It is a subject of immense practical relevance and importance to medical practitioners of all grades and specialities.

The ethical basis of legal consent

Ethical principles provide the basis of laws and regulations but are not enforceable. Laws and regulations provide an enforceable code giving rise to rights and remedies. The law on consent is based on the following related principles:

- desirability of self-determination
- respect for individual integrity.

The nature of consent

Consent consists of three separate but related elements: voluntariness, capacity and knowledge. Voluntariness means the willingness of the patient to undergo treatment. Capacity means that the patient is able to understand the nature of the treatment. Knowledge means that sufficient information as to the nature of the treatment has been disclosed to the patient. These three elements are *inter*dependent rather than independent. Legal consent requires all three elements to be present, and a failure of any one element can mean the failure of consent.

The legal consequences of lack of consent

The general principle is that consent is required for treatment. A procedure carried out on a patient without the patient's consent is *prima facie* an infringement of that patient's rights and may give rise to remedies in criminal and civil law. Criminal prosecutions are usually brought by the state and are punitive; civil actions are usually brought by the aggrieved individual and are compensatory. Criminal cases require the proof of criminal intent on the part of the doctor. *Bona fide* clinical treatment negates such criminality.

Tort: battery and negligence

Civil remedies arising from lack of consent give rise to actions in tort (a civil wrong). The two actions in tort are battery and negligence. Battery is the unlawful infliction of force upon another person. Negligence is the failure to take reasonable care. In tort the remedy is monetary damages. The purpose is compensatory; the damages awarded are intended to put the injured party in the position he would have been in had the tort not been committed.

The question arises as to whether an action for battery or negligence or both is appropriate where there has been a failure of consent. It is the failure of any of the elements of voluntariness, capacity or knowledge which gives rise to an action in battery or negligence as the case may be. A failure of voluntariness gives rise to an action in battery. A failure of knowledge, which can be formulated as a breach of the duty to inform, gives rise to an action in negligence.

THE LAW ON CONSENT IN MEDICAL PRACTICE

The law on consent to medical treatment conveniently divides into three separate parts according to the age of the patients concerned: adults, children of 16 and 17 years, and children under 16 years.

Adults

The recent case law on consent involving competent adults has generally concerned claims where there is an allegation of failure to inform. The claims are accordingly founded in negligence rather than battery. The duty to inform is part of the bundle of duties that arises from the therapeutic relationship.

The legal standard which determines liability in medical negligence is the 'Bolam' test:[1] a doctor was not guilty of negligence if he acted in accordance with a practice accepted as proper by a responsible body of medical men skilled in that particular art.

The duty of a doctor was to explain what he intended to do and its implications in accordance with the standards of a careful and responsible doctor in similar circumstances; there was no duty to canvass anything other than the inherent implications of the treatment; the fundamental assumption was that the doctor knew his job and would do it properly and ought only to warn of a real risk, taking into account the personality of the patient, the risk and the nature of the warning.[2]

The application of the Bolam test with respect to the duty to inform was examined by the House of Lords.[3] The court examined two different doctrines of the standard and extent of disclosure of the duty to inform. The plaintiff argued that the doctrine of informed consent should apply; the defendant argued that the Bolam test should apply. The majority of the House favoured the Bolam test. The application of the Bolam test has been criticised as allowing the medical profession to determine the legal standard of medical practice. The court, however, qualified the Bolam test: the court was not bound to accept the medical evidence as conclusive. It was a rule of evidence rather than a rule of law. Lord Scarman, however, favoured the doctrine of informed consent and set it out in his dissenting speech: where there was a real or material risk inherent in the proposed treatment the question as to whether the patient should be warned and the extent of the warning was to be considered in accordance with the right of self-determination. Accordingly, the patient should be informed of the inherent risk irrespective of the medical practice. The materiality of a risk was to be determined by reference to a hypothetical prudent patient. Lord Scarman recognised, however, that informed consent was subject to an overriding therapeutic privilege: if the information concerning the risk was detrimental to the health of the patient then it need not be disclosed.

---

1 *Bolam v Friern Hospital Management Committee* [1957] 1 WLR 582
2 *Chatterton v Gerson and Another* [1981] QB 432
3 *Sidaway v Governors of Bethlem Royal Hospital and the Maudsley Hospital* (HL) [1985] AC 871

Children

The general principle is that parents have the right to give consent on behalf of their children. This is derived from the old common law rule that parents had control over their children. Such a rule has been largely displaced by the change in attitudes of modern society. The principle now is that the welfare of the child is the paramount consideration. Accordingly, the exercise of consent by parents on behalf of their children is for the benefit of the children. The parents' rights are not absolute and where, for instance, the welfare of children is at risk, such rights may be exercised by a local authority in respect of children in care. Ultimately, the welfare of children is protected by the courts. Children can be conveniently divided into those 16 years and older and those younger.

Children of 16 years and older

Children of 16 years or more are to be regarded as though they were adults for the purposes of consent. The Family Law Reform Act 1969 provides at section 8(1):

The consent of a minor who has attained the age of sixteen years to any surgical, medical or dental treatment which, in the absence of consent, would constitute a trespass to his person, shall be as effective as it would be if he were of full age; and where a minor has by virtue of this section given an effective consent to any treatment it shall not be necessary to obtain any consent for it from his parent or guardian.

This provision affects only the position of those who come within its scope and leaves unaffected the position of those who do not. It is confined to consent and is not concerned with refusal (see below). Thus, the consent of an incompetent minor of 16 or 17 is covered by common law. Similarly, the consent of children under the age of 16 is covered by common law.

Children under 16 years

A child has the right to make his own decision upon sufficient maturity to understand the nature of the matter requiring decision.[4] 'Gillick competence' imports the notion of a child having sufficient understanding and intelligence to enable him to understand fully what is proposed and its consequences in order to give consent.

---

4 *Gillick* v *West Norfolk and Wisbech Area Health Authority and Another* (HL) [1986] AC 112

The assessment of 'Gillick competence' is a matter for the doctor in his clinical judgment of the individual patient. 'Gillick competence' thus recognises the right of self-determination of young persons and acknowledges that parental rights over children are dwindling and can be overridden. They are residual and are only wholly extinguished at the age of majority.

The notion of 'Gillick competence' is confined to consent and does not apply to refusal (see below).

TREATMENT OF MENTAL DISORDER

There is no common law principle that because a patient is suffering from some form of mental disorder a doctor may treat him without his consent. Unless clear statutory authority to the contrary exists no-one may be detained in a hospital or to undergo medical treatment or even to be submitted to a medical examination without his consent; this is as true of a mentally disordered person as anyone else.

Under the scheme of the Mental Health Act 1983 (see Ch. 5) Parliament created statutory powers whereby the mentally disordered may be detained for treatment of their mental disorder (but not other conditions) under compulsion; actions may not be brought against any persons exercising such powers unless it is shown that the person has failed to act in good faith or with reasonable care. Notwithstanding such statutory powers enabling patients to be involuntarily detained and treated, it is good practice for consent to be obtained whenever possible.

The Act defines mental disorder as mental illness, arrested or incomplete development of mind, psychopathic disorder or disability of mind.

MENTAL INCAPACITY IN ADULTS

The question of consent of adult patients lacking capacity is governed by statute and common law. The Mental Health Act 1983 is limited in its scope to treatment of mental disorder of certain defined categories of patients. The position regarding treatment of such patients for conditions other than mental disorders, or any medical treatment of patients outside such defined categories, is governed by common law.

The law concerning the treatment of adult patients permanently lacking capacity (i.e. mentally handicapped) for conditions other than mental disorder was, until recently, unclear. In *Re F*,[5] the court recognised it had no jurisdiction either to give or to withhold consent to treatment. The court, however, had inherent jurisdiction to examine the lawfulness of such treatment and to make a declaration to that effect. The court recognised that in some cases it was the medical duty to treat, and acknowledged that for many years this was the medical practice.

The court was anxious to lay down some common law principles to determine the lawfulness or otherwise of such treatment: treatment was lawful if it was in the 'best interests' of the patient. Treatment was in the 'best interests' if, but only if, it was carried out either to save life or to ensure improvement or to prevent deterioration in physical or mental health. The question of 'best interests' should be determined in accordance with the Bolam principle. The practicalities of the medical care of the mentally incapacitated were appreciated by the court; such treatment included emergency major surgery as well as routine nursing procedures. The court implicitly recognised a sliding scale of medical autonomy according to the seriousness of the medical intervention. Thus, routine minor procedures would present no difficulties. In respect of more serious treatment, it was desirable and good practice to consult relatives. In some cases a number of specialists would need to be consulted and, in cases involving more than a purely medical opinion, an interdisciplinary approach would be appropriate. The court's opinion should be sought as to the lawfulness of an operation as serious as sterilization; this practice should extend to other operations and procedures which, although therapeutic, contain a large element of social policy in their indication.

WITHDRAWAL OF TREATMENT

The doctrine of 'best interests' was examined in a case concerning withdrawal of treatment, *Airedale NHS Trust* v *Bland*.[6] The court held that the object of medical treatment and care was to benefit the patient; since a large body of informed and responsible medical opinion considered that the persistent vegetative state was not a benefit to the patient, the principle of the sanctity

5 *Re F (Mental Patient: Sterilisation)* (HL) [1990] 2 AC
6 *Airedale NHS Trust* v *Bland* (HL) [1993] 2 WLR 317

of life, which was not absolute, was not violated by ceasing to give medical treatment to which the patient had not consented and which conferred no benefit upon him. The doctors responsible for the patient were neither under a duty nor entitled to continue such medical treatment since the patient had no further interest in being kept alive. Until a body of experience and practice had been built up it was desirable that an application should be made to court in any case where medical staff considered that continued treatment of a patient in a persistent vegetative state no longer conferred benefit upon him; this was in the interests of the protection of patients and doctors, the reassurance of patients' families and that of the public. The court stated that the moral, social and legal issues of the case should be considered by Parliament.

REFUSAL OF TREATMENT: ADULTS

A competent adult has an absolute right to refuse treatment for reasons which are rational, irrational, unknown or even non-existent. The court has advised that doctors should consider the true scope and basis of the refusal; further, they should give careful consideration to the patient's capacity to make the decision and whether it was an independent decision. In cases of doubt as to the effect of a purported refusal of treatment, where failure to treat seriously threatened the health of the patient, doctors should apply to the courts for guidance.[7]

The court has recently granted a declaration that the operation of caesarean section and necessary consequential treatment was in the vital interests of a mother and her unborn child and could be lawfully performed despite the refusal of the mother.[8] The mother was in arrested labour and her condition was desperately serious; her refusal could not be questioned. The court held, however, that there was no authority directly on this point and, accordingly, granted the declaration. This dictum appears inconsistent with earlier guidelines set out by the Court of Appeal.[9] which stated that it was not for the judiciary to extend the law in such circumstances. It was a matter for Parliament.

---

7 *Re T (Adult: Medical Treatment)* [1992] 3 WLR 782
8 *Re S (Adult: Refusal of Treatment)* [1992] 3 WLR 806
9 *Re F (in utero)* [1988] Fam 122

REFUSAL OF TREATMENT: CHILDREN UNDER 16 YEARS

The court has power to consent to medical treatment of a child under 16 who is competent to consent to treatment but who has refused or was not asked; conversely, the court has an overriding power which natural parents do not have, to refuse consent or forbid treatment even if the child consents, if the consent or refusal of consent by the court is in the child's interest.[10] The court considered the distinction between consent and refusal: no doctor could be required to treat a child save in accordance with his professional judgment; there could be concurrent powers to consent, each of which was enabling; refusal of treatment was only effective if all having such powers were unanimous; a 'Gillick competent' child shared the power to consent with his parent or guardian; 'Gillick competence' was a developmental concept which took into consideration mental disability; the court could override the decisions of a 'Gillick competent' child and his parents.

REFUSAL OF TREATMENT: CHILDREN OF 16 AND OLDER

The court in the exercise of its inherent jurisdiction over minors held that the refusal (or consent) of a child of 16 years could be overridden if it was in her best interests.[11] The court stated also that parents (or, for children in care, the local authority) could override such refusal, though not consent. Section 8(1) of the Family Law Reform Act 1969 was considered; it was concerned with consent and not refusal. The express purpose was to provide a defence to trespass so that older children could give consent on their own behalf. The section was not concerned with self-determination of older children. The concurrent power of consent of parents was expressly preserved.

REFUSAL OF TREATMENT: SUMMARY

In summary and as a general rule, the legal effect of refusal is the same as the absence of consent (save in the case of the emergency treatment of unconscious adults). In competent adults there is only one power of consent or refusal, which resides in that adult and is, therefore, determinative.

---

10 *Re R (A Minor) (Wardship: Medical Treatment)* (CA) [1992] Fam 11
11 *Re W (A Minor) (Inherent Jurisdiction: Consent to Treatment)* [1992] 3 WLR 758

With children there are concurrent powers of consent and refusal. Whereas the child's consent is enabling, his refusal is not disabling (because consent may be exercised by another). This asymmetry between the effects of consent and refusal is strictly logical and internally consistent but conflicts with the principle of self-determination for minors and the spirit of the Children Act 1989.

For incompetent minors and incompetent adults a refusal of treatment is not determinative; if such persons cannot give valid consent, then they cannot give valid refusal. Obviously, their wishes are a factor to be taken into consideration.

EMERGENCY TREATMENT

There may be circumstances where the medical indication for rapid intervention overrides the requirement to obtain consent. Examples include the unconscious adult patient. Emergency treatment without consent has been considered by the court in *Gillick*. Its lawfulness was assumed and subsequent approval, if required, would be granted where appropriate. Such treatment is to be administered in accordance with the 'best interest' principle. A conservative approach should be adopted and only necessary procedures should be carried out; what could be carried out electively should be deferred. It could then be discussed with the patient. This accords with the prudent clinical practice of performing limited emergency procedures and confining medical treatments to elective procedures where possible.

Third party proxy

It is a common medical practice to seek 'consent' from relatives in cases where an adult is unable to give consent for treatment. Third party consent is generally of no legal effect in the case of adults, whether competent or incompetent. It is, however, good practice to consult relatives and others concerned with the care of the patient. This provides an opportunity to counsel them and to take their wishes into consideration. The management of the patient, however, is determined in accordance with the doctrine of 'best interests'.

CONSENT FORMS

The use of consent forms is universal in medical practice. The consent form is not to be equated with consent itself, but is merely evidence of consent. Thus, procedures may be carried out without true consent where there is a completed consent form, and, conversely, procedures may be carried with consent where there is not a completed consent form. Consent forms are usually only evidence as to the voluntariness of the procedure; they are not usually evidence of the discharge of the duty to inform, although increasingly elaborate consent forms are being devised. Most consent forms are not limited to any named procedure but contain verbal formulae extending the procedure to what is necessary and in the best interests of the patient and can be medically justified should unforeseen circumstances arise.

CONCLUSION

Ethical principles provide the basis of an enforceable code protecting the individual's personal rights. Recent case law has provided guidelines for medical practice, converting ethical principles into legal rules. This process is not absolute and the courts have identified the limitations of the law and acknowledged the contribution of the ethics of medical practice. Lord Goff observed in *Bland* at page 374:[6]

The truth is that, in the course of their work, doctors frequently have to make decisions which may affect the continued survival of their patients, and are in reality far more experienced in matters of this kind than are the judges. It is nevertheless the function of the judges to state the legal principles upon which the lawfulness of the actions of doctors depend; but in the end the decisions to be made in individual cases must rest with the doctors themselves. In these circumstances, what is required is a sensitive understanding by both the judges and the doctors of each other's respective functions, and in particular a determination by the judges not merely to understand the problems facing the medical profession in cases of this kind, but also to regard their professional standards with respect. Mutual understanding between the doctors and the judges is the best way to ensure the evolution of a sensitive and sensible framework for the treatment and care of patients, with a sound ethical base, in the interest of the patients themselves.

Clinicians need to be acquainted with both ethics and law; an understanding of consent issues is, therefore, a necessary requirement of the medical practitioner's clinical competence.

FURTHER READING

Jones M 1995 Medical negligence (2nd edn). Sweet & Maxwell, London
Kennedy I, Grubb A 1994 Medical law (2nd edn). Butterworths, London
Powers M, Harris N 1994 Medical negligence (2nd edn). Butterworths, London

5. The Mental Health Act (England and Wales)

Alain Gregoire

The Mental Health Act 1983 relates to issues of consent to treatment and admission of mentally disordered people in England and Wales. This Act of Parliament is divided into 10 parts (Box 5.1) and 149 sections. Only a few of these are immediately relevant to common clinical practice and these will be considered in this chapter. For the purposes of the Act, mental disorder is divided into three broad categories:

1. Mental illness: not specifically defined but promiscuity, immorality, sexual deviancy and alcohol abuse are specifically excluded.
2. Mental impairment or severe mental impairment: defined in terms of impairment of intelligence and social function when associated with abnormally aggressive or seriously irresponsible conduct.
3. Psychopathic disorder: persistent disorder or disability of mind which results in abnormally aggressive or seriously irresponsible conduct (with or without impairment of intelligence).

Box 5.1 The 10 parts of the Mental Health Act 1983

Part I: Defines mental disorder
Part II: Civil Detention Orders and Guardianship
Part III: Criminal Justice Orders
Part IV: Consent to treatment
Part V: Mental Health Tribunals
Part VI: Movement of patients in and out of England and Wales
Part VII: Court of Protection
Part VIII: Duties of local authorities and the Secretary of State
Part IX: Offences
Part X: Miscellaneous provisions

THE MENTAL HEALTH ACT COMMISSION

The Mental Health Act Commission is a statutory body appointed by the Secretary of State to oversee and regulate the correct application of the Act. The Commission consists of a panel of psychiatrists, nurses, social workers, lawyers and members of the lay public under the chairmanship of a lawyer. Their duties include preparing a Code of Practice,[a] visiting all psychiatric hospitals and registered mental nursing homes, scrutinising documents relating to the detention of patients under the Act and investigating complaints. They appoint second opinion approved doctors (SOADs — see Box 5.2). They are now also involved in overseeing the proper application of supervision registers and the care programme approach.

Box 5.2 Glossary

ASW: Approved Social Worker — qualified to make applications for detention under the Act

MHAC: Mental Health Act Commission

MHRT: Mental Health Review Tribunal

RMO: Responsible Medical Officer — Doctor (consultant) in charge of patient's care

Section 12(2) Approved Doctor: Doctor with experience of psychiatry and approved by the Region to make medical recommendations under the Act

SOAD: Second Opinion Approved Doctor — psychiatrist appointed by MHAC

Civil Detention Orders

These include the longer term treatment orders (Sections 3 and 7) and the briefer orders for assessment (Sections 2, 4, 5, 135, 136).

Section 2: Admission for assessment

This allows compulsory admission for up to 28 days, for assessment or assessment followed by treatment for mental disorder. This order is appropriate when the patient is not well known to the service or when the diagnosis or most appropriate management are not established. The formalities involve application by the patient's nearest relative or preferably an Approved Social Worker (ASW), supported by two medical recommendations. The latter *must* include at least one section 12 approved doctor and one doctor with previous acquaintance of the patient (usually the patient's general practitioner); if this is not possible it is desirable for both doctors to be section 12 approved. The following grounds must apply:

1. The patient is suffering from a mental disorder of a nature or degree which warrants such detention **and** the admission is necessary in the interests of the patient's own health **or** safety **or** for the protection of others.

2. The ASW and doctors should also satisfy themselves that alternative forms of care or treatment, including informal admission, are not possible. They have a professional responsibility to ensure that they obtain as much information as possible about the patient and that they discuss the patient with each other. It is the doctors' responsibility to ensure that a hospital bed will be available. Admission to hospital must take place within 14 days of the completion of the latest medical recommendation. No more than 5 days must elapse between the doctors' examinations of the patient.

Section 2 cannot be renewed. If continued detention is necessary Section 3 should be considered.

Section 4: Emergency admission for assessment

This allows compulsory admission for up to 72 hours for assessment and should only be used in emergency situations in the community when the delay in obtaining a second opinion for a section 2 admission would result in a significant risk of harm to the patient or others, or serious harm to property. Only one medical recommendation from a registered medical practitioner is required. Application can be made by nearest relative or preferably by an ASW. The latter must satisfy himself that the situation is a genuine emergency and that there are adequate grounds for proceeding without a second doctor. The convenience of any of those involved does not constitute adequate grounds. Both the applicant and the doctor must have seen the patient within the previous 24 hours and the doctor should preferably know the patient. Admission must take place within 24 hours of completion of the earliest form.

Unlike sections 2 and 3, this Section does not allow for compulsory treatment (except under common law).

A second medical opinion must be obtained as soon as possible with a view to converting to a section 2. Social Services should be informed of this, although the original ASW application remains valid. The section 2 is then valid for 28 days from when the section 4 took effect.

Section 5: Detention of informal inpatients

This allows for the emergency detention of an informal inpatient in a hospital or registered nursing home for the purposes of an assessment with a view to a section 2 or 3. Section 5(4) is the nurse's holding power which may be used by a registered mental health nurse if a registered medical practitioner is not immediately available. This has a maximum duration of 6 hours and expires upon arrival of the Responsible Medical Officer's (RMO's) nominated deputy who should attend as soon as possible. Section 5(2) may be used by the RMO's nominated deputy to detain an informal inpatient, or an inpatient held under section 5(4) for the purposes of an assessment. This section has a maximum duration of 72 hours. However, it should not be allowed to expire as an assessment should have been carried out prior to that time. The section 5(2) ceases to apply from the moment that assessment has been completed and the patient therefore becomes informal unless another section of the Act is applied.

Section 135

Section 135 is a magistrate's warrant allowing an ASW entry to a private residence to remove a person thought to be suffering from a mental disorder and who has been, or is being, ill-treated, neglected or kept otherwise than under proper control **or** is unable to care for himself and is living alone. The person is conveyed to a place of safety for up to 72 hours for the purpose of an assessment by a registered medical practitioner and ASW.

Section 136: Mentally disordered persons found in public places

Section 136 allows a police officer to remove to a place of safety any person who appears to be suffering from a mental disorder in a place to which the public has access. The person must appear to be in immediate need of care and control and such action must appear necessary in the person's interest or for the protection of others. A maximum of 72 hours is allowed, during which the person **must** be assessed by an ASW **and** a registered medical practitioner. Local policy must be agreed between Social Services, Health Services and the police in all areas.

Section 3: Admission for treatment

Under section 3, compulsory admission is allowed for **up to** 6 months for treatment. The same requirements for medical recommendations apply as for section 2. Application can be made by nearest relative or (preferably) by an ASW who must make every effort to contact the nearest relative. The ASW cannot proceed with the application if the nearest relative objects. However, a County Court can transfer the powers of the nearest relative if it considers the objection to be unreasonable. The following grounds must apply:

1. The patient is suffering from a mental illness, severe mental illness, psychopathic disorder or mental impairment; one of these categories must be specified and agreed by both doctors and applicant **and**
2. The mental disorder is of a degree which makes it appropriate for the patient to receive treatment in hospital **and**
3. It is necessary in the interests of his health **or** safety **or** for the protection of others that he receive such treatment and it cannot be provided unless he is detained, **and**
4. In the case of mental impairment or psychopathic disorder, such treatment is likely to alleviate or prevent a deterioration in his condition. The same time limits as for section 2 apply to the completion of documents. Section 3 is renewable by the RMO for 6 months in the first instance, then yearly if the grounds for admission continue to apply.

Section 7: Guardianship

Under section 7 a guardian, normally the local authority social services department, is empowered to require the patient to:

1. live at a specified place
2. attend for outpatient treatment, occupation, education or

training (although there is no power to enforce cooperation or compliance with such interventions)

3.   permit access to himself at the place where he is living.

Requirements for application are as for section 3 and the patient must be 16 years of age or over. Duration and renewal is as for section 3.

Unless the patient recognises the authority of the Guardian and as a result cooperates with the Guardian, this Order conveys little benefit. The Code of Practice states that if there is consistent lack of compliance the Order should be discharged. The Order is little used, and it is debatable whether it is under-used.

PATIENTS CONCERNED IN CRIMINAL PROCEEDINGS (PART 3 OF THE ACT)

Patients awaiting trial

Section 35 allows the remand of an accused person to hospital for a report for 28 days, renewable for up to 12 weeks. One medical recommendation from a section 12 approved doctor is required, in addition to a court order. Crown Courts may apply this order to any person awaiting trial for an imprisonable offence. In magistrates' courts the person must be convicted or awaiting sentencing, or the court must be satisfied that he committed the act or made the omission **or** he must consent to the exercise of the power.

Section 36: Remand to hospital for treatment

Section 36 permits a Crown Court accompanied by two medical recommendations (one of them by an approved doctor) to remand an accused person to hospital for treatment for up to 28 days renewable for up to 12 weeks.

Convicted offenders

Section 37: Hospital admission or Guardianship Order

This provides the court with an alternative to imprisonment or other punishment and has the same effect as applying a section 3 or Guardianship Order. Once it is implemented the Court has no further involvement with the patient. The Order requires that the same grounds as for section 3 apply to the patient **and** that the court is satisfied that this is the most suitable method of disposing of the case **and** that the court has two medical recommendations (one from an approved doctor) and, in the case of a hospital order, that the hospital has agreed to admit the patient.

Section 48:

The Home Secretary also has the power to transfer such persons to hospital when urgent treatment is required. A Restriction Order (see below) is applied for people detained in prison on remand.

Section 38: Interim hospital order

Under Section 38 two medical recommendations are required (one from an approved doctor **and** one from the admitting hospital) that the person is suffering from mental illness, psychopathic disorder, severe mental impairment or mental impairment such that the hospital order may be appropriate **and** that he will be admitted within 28 days. This can be converted to a section 37 by the Court at any stage.

Section 47: Home Secretary's power to transfer sentenced prisoners

Section 47 allows the Home Secretary, on the basis of two written medical recommendations (one from an approved doctor) to transfer a convicted offender to hospital. The doctors must agree on the form of mental disorder as for section 3. The Home Secretary can order the person back to prison at any time.

Restricted Detention Orders

Section 41: Order restricting discharge

Such an order is applied in addition to section 37 (Section 37/41) by a Crown Court after considering:

- the nature of the offence
- antecedents of the offender
- risk of further offences
- protection of the public

The Court must have heard oral evidence from at least one of the medical practitioners. The Restriction Order has the effect of giving the Home Secretary the responsibility for granting leave and allowing discharge with or without limit of time. The RMO must request permission from the Home Secretary for any leave (except within hospital grounds), transfer or discharge. The Hospital Order (Section 37) does not expire or require renewal while the section 41 is in force. Patients can be conditionally discharged, the section 41 remaining in place, and must abide by conditions imposed by the Home Office. Breaking conditions can lead to readmission under Section 37/41. Informal admission of section 41 patients is also possible.

Section 49: Restriction of prisoners transferred to hospital

Section 49 has the same effect as Section 41 but is applied to Section 47 (Section 47/49). This can be terminated at any time by the Home Secretary and expires when the fixed term of the prisoner's sentence ends. Applications can be made to the Home Secretary for discharge.

PART IV OF THE ACT: CONSENT TO TREATMENT

Part IV applies to patients detained under all sections of the Act **except** sections 4, 5(4), 5(2), 135, 136, patients in a place of safety under section 37 pending admission to hospital, and patients subject to section 7 (guardianship). The provisions allow for the administration of reversible medical treatments (medication or electroconvulsive therapy (ECT)) without consent for up to 3 months to patients detained under a section to which this part applies. However, consent must first be sought in all patients. The provisions apply only to medical treatment for mental disorder. Treatment of physical disorder can only lawfully be given under the Act if this is necessary to alleviate the mental disorder.

Section 57: Treatments requiring the patient's consent **and** a second opinion (from a SOAD)

This applies at present only to psychosurgery and surgical hormone implantation to reduce male sex-drive. This safeguard applies also to informal patients.

Section 58: Treatments requiring consent **or** a second opinion

Section 58 applies to patients who have been treated with medication for 3 months (with or without consent) and to any detained

patient requiring ECT. Consent must be certified by the RMO or
section 12 approved doctor, or a SOAD must agree to the treatment
plan.

Section 62

In urgent situations, when immediately necessary, reversible treatments may be given without consent under the direction of the
RMO.

Section 63

A range of therapeutic interventions are covered by section 63,
such as nursing care, occupational therapy or behaviour therapy for
which consent should be sought but is not required. However, such
interventions are unlikely to be particularly effective without some
degree of cooperation.

PART V: RIGHTS OF APPEAL

Hospital managers have a duty to inform patients of their rights
verbally and in writing at the beginning of a compulsory admission: these include information about the detention order, consent
to treatment, rights of appeal and complaints procedures. Rights of
appeal and nearest relative's rights are summarised in Table 5.1.
Patients detained under sections 2, 3 or 37 may appeal to the managers as often as they wish.

Table 5.1 Rights of appeal to Mental Health Review Tribunals

Section	Rights of appeal	
	By patient	By nearest relative
Section 2	within 14 days	none
Section 3*	to MHRT — in first 6 months	none
Guardianship	to MHRT — in first 6 months	none
Section 37**	after 6 months, then yearly	after 6 months, then yearly
Section 37/41	after 6 months, then yearly	none

* Automatic appeal after 6 months without an MHRT hearing, and 3-yearly thereafter
** Automatic appeal after 3 years' detention without an MHRT hearing

NB: Patients detained under Sections 2, 3 & 37 may appeal to Hospital Managers as
often as they wish.

Conclusions and future developments

The Mental Health Act 1983 provides the legal framework for the difficult balancing act between the basic human and civil rights of mentally ill individuals on the one hand, and on the other their right to receive treatment for severe mental illness and the need to protect them and other members of society from the effects of such illness[b,c,d]. The use of the Mental Health Act should never replace attempts to gain patients' cooperation with treatment through the development of good relations, discussion, education, persuasion, compromise and bargaining. Failure to explore adequate alternative forms of management goes against the spirit of the Act.

Mental Health services in the United Kingdom have undergone a considerable shift of emphasis from inpatient care to care outside hospitals. However, the Mental Health Act 1983 is almost entirely hospital-focused and it has become increasingly apparent that the Act fails to meet the needs of patients and professionals in the community setting.[e] Community treatment orders have been proposed, which would allow enforced treatment in the community of patients satisfying strict criteria.[f,g]. This has been opposed as an infringement of human rights,[h] but it is arguable that the current situation, which involves enforced treatment combined with hospitalisation, is a greater infringement, particularly in the case of patients who only require the treatment and not necessarily the hospitalisation.

The Mental Health (Patients in the Community) Act 1995 gives key workers (normally CPNs) new powers in the community, including the power to require patients to live in a specified place and attend for treatment, and to seek the RMO's review with a view to recall to hospital if they fail to comply with medication.

Such measures have been criticised as introducing or even imposing coercive practices on professionals without giving them adequate power simply to treat patients.[i] This legislative change will be occurring in the context of other contractual developments in mental health services including the Care Programme Approach (CPA),[j] which provides a formalised framework for the management of all patients in contact with NHS mental health services, and the Supervision Register[k] which was established by the Department of Health following the Clunis inquiry.[l]

Community care offers considerable benefits to the majority of individuals with mental illness through flexible, needs-led approaches to management combined with effective systems for assessing those needs and delivering and monitoring care. However, an important minority of patients with chronic symptoms remain disturbed, vulnerable and occasionally dangerous, and require very considerable resources which may not always be available. Thus we continue to see the appalling personal and social consequences of severe mental illness, and the resulting media coverage leads to dramatic criticisms of community care and demands for greater legislative powers to control the mentally ill.

REFERENCES

a   Department of Health and Welsh Office 1993 Code of practice, Mental Health Act 1983. HMSO, London

b   Department of Health and Social Security 1983 Mental Health Act 1983. Memorandum on parts I–IV, VIII and X. HMSO, London

c   Gostin L 1983 A practical guide to mental health law. MIND, London

d   Royal Commission on the laws relating to mental illness and mental deficiencies. 1957 Report. HMSO, London

e   Turner T 1988 Community care. British Journal of Psychiatry 152: 1–3

f   Royal College of Psychiatrists 1987 Community treatment orders: a discussion document. Royal College of Psychiatrists, London

g   Royal College of Psychiatrists 1993 Community supervision orders. Royal College of Psychiatrists, London

h   House of Commons Health Committee 1993 Community supervision orders. Health Committee 5th report, volume 1. HMSO, London

i   Eastman N 1995 Anti-therapeutic community mental health law. British Medical Journal 310: 1081–1082

j   Department of Health 1990 Care programme approach. Health circular (90)23/local authority social services letter (90)11. 1994 Department of Health, London

k   Glover G R, MacCulloch A W, Jenkins R 1994 Supervision registers for mentally ill people. British Medical Journal 309: 809–810

l   Ritchie J, Dick D, Lingham R 1994 The report of the inquiry into the care and treatment of Christopher Clunis. HMSO, London

6. Confidentiality

Peter Schutte

INTRODUCTION

Ever since the Hippocratic Oath was first taken 2500 years ago, the medical profession has recognised confidentiality as a cornerstone of good clinical practice. In 1947, the Declaration of Geneva (amended in 1968) strongly reinforced the Hippocratic Oath. It states:

'I will respect the secrets which are confided in me, even after the patient has died.'

Yet in recent times, legal, social and technological advances and the emergence of Human Immunodeficiency Virus (HIV) infection have brought increasingly complex pressures to bear on healthcare professionals to breach professional confidentiality.

The courts give almost absolute protection to the confidence between a lawyer and his client. The law will not extend the same privilege to healthcare professionals, and a presiding officer of a court may, on occasions, direct a breach of medical confidentiality.

In contrast with countries such as France and Belgium, and with some limited exceptions, medical confidentiality is not protected by statutory law in the United Kingdom. Confidentiality may be enforced by a patient through an injunction or an action for damages in a civil court, but in the absence of any demonstrable harm, it is likely that the damages awarded would be nominal. Civil claims are therefore very rare.

All staff employed by the National Health Service (NHS) may be subjected to disciplinary proceedings following a breach of confidentiality, but for self-employed general medical practitioners, the duty of confidentiality *per se* falls outside their contractual obligations under the NHS Terms of Service.

In practical terms, it falls to registration bodies such as the General Medical Council (GMC), United Kingdom Central Council for Nursing, Midwifery and Health Visiting (UKCC) and the various boards of the Council for Professions Supplementary to Medicine to enforce medical confidentiality as an ethical rather than a legal matter. However, no-one should underestimate the consequences for a registered practitioner of a finding of serious professional misconduct arising from such a breach. His name could be erased from the Register, depriving him of his livelihood. And no-one should underestimate the vigour with which the registration bodies will pursue an allegation of breach of medical confidentiality.

The registration bodies publish guidelines on confidentiality and all registered practitioners should study these carefully and review them when they are updated.[a,b]

DISCLOSURE TO THE PATIENT

Anyone holding computerised information which includes 'personal data' is obliged under the Data Protection Act 1984 to supply a copy of that information to the individual concerned upon request.

The Access to Health Records Act 1990 came into force on 1 November 1991. A patient may obtain access to their own medical records made after that date. Clinical records made before then may be obtained compulsorily if the patient is, or may become, a plaintiff in civil proceedings, under the provisions of the Supreme Court Act 1981.

It is becoming common practice for practitioners to agree to the disclosure of all the clinical notes in their possession to a patient (or a patient's legal representative) on demand, although, subject to the statutory provisions set out above, no patient has an absolute right in law to see his medical records.[1] When a practitioner in person is the subject of a complaint or litigation, disclosure is usually carried out with the assistance of the practitioner's medical defence organisation. The consent of other practitioners who have written in the notes is not necessary.

All the relevant Acts of Parliament contain provisions for resisting the disclosure of information to the patient where, in the clinical judgment of the doctor in possession or control of the notes, disclosure may cause harm to the patient or cause a breach of confidentiality to a third party.

---

1 *R v Mid Glamorgan Family Health Service Authority & Others* [1994] 5 Med LR 383

Disclosure to third parties

Where a patient or a properly authorised representative gives consent to the disclosure of information to a third party, the practitioner may agree to do so in accordance with that consent. Where any doubt exists in the practitioner's mind about the validity of the consent, he has an obligation to clarify the issues with the patient.

Disclosure to a third party *contrary* to the patient's wishes should only take place in the most exceptional circumstances, for example where the health, safety or welfare of someone may otherwise be placed at serious risk.

Disclosure without the consent of the patient

Disclosure to relatives and others caring for the patient

Information is often shared with a patient's relatives or other persons helping to care for the patient. This may be without the patient's authority, but usually when the patient's consent is implied and only where it is in the patient's best medical interests to do so. This situation most frequently occurs with terminally ill patients.

Normally a practitioner will disclose all information concerning a young child to parents. Where parents are separated or divorced, information may still be disclosed to either parent unless a court has removed parental responsibility from one parent. It is important that where information is given to one parent's solicitors, the confidentiality of the other parent should not be compromised and this may be achieved by removing any information about the other parent before passing on the notes.

Children over 16 enjoy the same rights to confidentiality as adults. This right may be inferred from the provisions of the Family Law Reform Act 1969 which enables children of 16 and over to consent to medical treatment.

For patients under the age of 16 the practitioner may have to exercise his discretion. Where the child's maturity and understanding is sufficient to enable an appreciation of what is involved (i.e. the child is 'Gillick competent',[2] — see Ch. 4) the practitioner must take the child's own wishes into account. The practitioner should make every reasonable effort to persuade the child to involve the parents or guardians in, for example, consenting to dis-

---

2 *Gillick* v *West Norfolk and Wisbech Health Authority and Another* [1995] 3 WLR 830; [1986] 3 All ER 402; [1986] 1 AC Crim LR 113

closure, but if on rare occasions in the practitioner's judgment it is in the child's best interests, then disclosure of information to the parents or guardians may take place. If the practitioner decides to disclose information to a parent or legal guardian contrary to the child's wishes, then he should, with very rare exceptions, inform the child in advance of his intentions.

Disclosure to other healthcare professionals

Clinical information is normally shared by a practitioner with other healthcare professionals involved in the care of a particular patient without the patient's consent and on a 'need to know' basis. The doctor has a duty to be satisfied that all members of staff are aware of their obligation to preserve confidentiality.

A practitioner who is the subject of complaint is not entitled to have access to clinical notes made by a colleague relating to the care of the patient after the events giving rise to the complaint, without the consent of the patient.

Disclosure as a statutory requirement

Certain infectious diseases must be notified by a doctor under the Public Health (Control of Disease) Act 1984 and various regulations. HIV infection is not a notifiable disease.

Information concerning patients addicted to drugs scheduled in the Misuse of Drugs (Notification of and Supply to Addicts) Regulations 1985 must be notified by a doctor to the Chief Medical Officer at the Home Office.

A doctor or midwife present at a birth must notify the relevant authority within 36 hours, and a doctor treating a patient in a terminal illness must provide a Certificate of Death stating *inter alia* the cause of death (NHS Notification of Births & Deaths Regulations 1974). It is not lawful to omit conditions contributing to death, such as HIV infection, from the certificate, however distressing this may be for the relatives of a deceased person.

Under the Abortion Act 1967, a doctor terminating a pregnancy must notify this.

Disclosure to employers and insurance companies

The Access to Medical Reports Act 1988 provides that, when a patient exercises his rights, employers and insurance companies may not be shown a report by a doctor who has seen the patient for clinical purposes, until the patient has seen the report and commented on it and given consent for its disclosure. Where a doctor sees a patient for an employer or an insurance company to assess the patient's fitness to work or life expectancy, the doctor must make sure from the outset that the patient understands the purpose of the consultation and obtains in advance the patient's consent in writing. If this doctor has not also seen the patient for clinical purposes, the report falls outside the provisions of the Act.

Occupational physicians have dual loyalties, both to their patients and to their employers. Where a firm provides a clinical service as a 'perk' for employees, it should be understood by the employer that the practitioner owes the patient the usual obligation of confidentiality.

Disclosure to social services and the police

Where a registered practitioner has reason to suspect child abuse, he will have an ethical obligation to volunteer information to an appropriate authority, such as Social Services. Only in very rare circumstances, where a doctor feels it is in the infant patient's best medical interests, will the doctor withhold information. An example might be where the doctor hears a confession of child sexual abuse which occurred many years previously, where there is no possibility of the abuse continuing and where the victim has pleaded for confidentiality to be respected.

Information which is given should be provided on a strictly 'need to know' basis, and care must be taken not to breach unnecessarily the medical confidentiality of parents or other persons involved in the care of the patient.

The Road Traffic Act 1988 places a duty upon any person to tell the police on request the name and address of a driver of a vehicle who may have been injured and who is alleged to be guilty of an offence under the Act. However, such disclosure should not include clinical information.

A patient who commits an offence such as assault against a healthcare professional or his staff, forgoes a degree of confidentiality. Normally the fact that a patient is a patient, is of itself strictly confidential information, but this need not prevent a healthcare professional from seeking the protection of the police where necessary. Disclosure to the police should be limited to the minimum necessary for the protection of the practitioner and his colleagues.

There is no legal obligation on any citizen to *volunteer* information to the police concerning a crime. An exception to this involves terrorism, which is defined as 'the use of violence for political ends' and includes 'any use of violence for the purposes of putting the public or any section of the public in fear'.

There are circumstances, albeit rare, where a breach of confidentiality may be justified on the grounds that failure to do so may place the patient or some other person at risk of serious harm or death.

In the case of *Tarasoff* v *Regents of University of California*[3] a psychiatrist was successfully sued after he had failed to warn the girlfriend of one of his patients that he knew her life was in danger. The patient later murdered the girl. No similar case has occurred in the UK and it is a matter of debate whether the UK courts would take the same view.

However, in the case of *W* v *Egdell* [1989][4] a claim was brought for damages against a UK consultant psychiatrist. He had examined a violent patient who was hoping to be released from detention under the Mental Health Act 1983, at the request of the patient's solicitors. The psychiatrist was so concerned by his findings that he disclosed a copy of his report to the appropriate authorities without the consent of the patient. As a consequence, the patient's application for release was turned down. A judge dismissed the claim and his decision was upheld by the Court of Appeal on the grounds that the doctor had acted in the public interest.

A healthcare professional may not necessarily be able to justify the voluntary disclosure of medical information to the police in relation to serious crime, particularly if the crime is non-violent or if the suspect is already in custody. Refusal by a healthcare professional to answer questions need not obstruct the police in their enquiries. Where the police require medical information to help convict a suspect, it is open to them to apply to a circuit judge for a court order under the Police and Criminal Evidence Act 1984, making the disclosure of medical information obligatory.

Doctors providing medical services for the police (forensic physicians) may find themselves in a particularly difficult situation arising from their dual role as personal clinicians to prisoners in a police cell on the one hand, and gatherers of forensic evidence for

---

3 Tarasoff v Regents of the University of California, 529 P 2d 5S (Cal, 1974); 551 P
   2d 334 (Cal, 1976)
4 W v Egdell [1990] 1 All ER 835, 849

the police on the other hand.[c] Their duty of medical confidentiality to a prisoner is no different from that of any other doctor to his patient. Forensic physicians should consider carefully any proposed contractual obligation placed on them by an employing police authority to disclose their clinical records as a matter of routine to police personnel without the prior and informed consent of the prisoner. This can be important because some prisoners may be drunk, under the influence of drugs, or psychotic, for example, and be unfit to give or withhold consent to the disclosure of information to the police at the time they are seen.

However, in such circumstances, the forensic physician does have a contractual obligation to tell the police if the prisoner is fit to be detained, fit to be interviewed and fit for trial, and also to provide such medical information as will enable the police to care properly for the prisoner, in the prisoner's best medical interests.

Disclosure to the Courts

A healthcare professional who is asked to breach confidentiality in a court of law must ask the judge or presiding officer for permission to breach confidentiality, but if directed to answer a question, may be found in contempt of court if he fails to do so and face a fine or imprisonment. A healthcare professional may be summoned to court and compelled to produce confidential documents subject to the judge's directions.

Disclosure to the Coroner

A healthcare professional normally requires the consent of a deceased patient's executors, or where the patient died intestate, the next of kin, before disclosing information. However, the coroner has powers to investigate the circumstance of a death, and clinical notes and relevant information should be disclosed to the coroner or coroner's officer to enable the coroner to determine whether an inquest should be held.

Disclosure for medical teaching, research, audit and administration

Medical information for use in teaching, research and audit is normally anonymised to preserve confidentiality. Where it may be possible to identify an individual, the patient concerned should be made aware of the possibility and given the opportunity to withhold consent to disclosure.

Where medical information identifiable to an individual is disclosed for administrative purposes, the healthcare professional should be satisfied that administrative staff are aware of their own duty of confidentiality, whether such staff work within the NHS or not.

CONCLUSION

The different priorities of medicine and the law make it difficult to resolve all of the problems which can arise from medical confidentiality. Healthcare professionals in doubt whether or not to disclose information without a patient's consent should not hesitate to contact their medical defence organisation or professional association for expert advice. The future is unlikely to see a simplification of the ethical or legal issues, and integration with Europe is likely to increase rather than decrease controversy in the UK. The Department of Health has issued detailed guidelines on medical confidentiality within the NHS,[d] and a working party including the British Medical Association has published a draft Bill[e] which would, if it became law, criminalise a wilful breach of confidentiality.

REFERENCES

a   General Medical Council 1995 Duties of a doctor: confidentiality. Guidance
    from the General Medical Council. General Medical Council, London
b   United Kingdom Central Council for Nursing, Midwifery and Health Visiting
    1992 Code of professional ethics for the nurse, midwife and health visitor,
    3rd edn. UKCC, London
c   Schutte P K 1993 Medical confidentiality and the police — GMC ruling. Journal
    of the Medical Defence Union 3:63
d   Department of Health 1996 Guidance on confidentiality, use and disclosure of
    personal health information. Department of Health, London
e   Multi-disciplinary Professional Working Group (including the British Medical
    Association) 1994 A Bill governing use and disclosure of personal health infor-
    mation. Available through the British Medical Association, Tavistock Square,
    London WC1H 9JP

FURTHER READING

Brazier M 1992 Medicine, patients and the law, 2nd edn. Penguin, London

British Medical Association 1993 Medical ethics today: its practice and philosophy. British Medical Association, London

Hoyte P J 1993 Can I see the records? Medical Defence Union, London

Mason J K, McCall Smith A 1994 Law and medical ethics, 4th edn. Butterworths, London

Medical Defence Union 1990 AIDS: Medico-legal advice. Medical Defence Union, London

O'Donovan C 1992 Confidentiality. Medical Defence Union, London

7. Death certification and the role of the coroner

Peter Dean

Historical development

It is in the general interests of the community that any sudden, unnatural or unexplained deaths should be investigated. To reflect this, the role of the coroner has evolved over the eight centuries since the office was formally established in 1194, from being a form of medieval tax gatherer to an independent judicial officer charged with the investigation of sudden, violent or unnatural death.

The duties of the early coroners were varied, and included the investigation of almost any aspect of medieval life that had the potential benefit of revenue for the Crown. Suicides were investigated, on the grounds that the goods and chattels of those found guilty of the crime of 'felo de se' or 'self murder' would then be forfeit to the crown, as were wrecks of the sea, fires, both fatal and non-fatal, and any discovery of buried treasure in the community, which is still on the statute books today as 'treasure trove'. Sudden death in the community had always been considered important and was also investigated, although for reasons far different from those of today.

After the Norman Conquest, to deter the local communities from a continuing habit of killing Normans, a heavy fine was levied on any village where a dead body was discovered, on the assumption that it was presumed to be Norman, unless it could be proved to be English. The fine was known as the 'Murdrum' (from which the word 'murder' is derived) and, as the system developed, many of the early coroners' inquests dealt with the 'Presumption of Normanry' which could only be rebutted by the local community, and a fine thus avoided, by the 'Presentment of Englishry'.

The coroner system continued to adapt over the centuries, but in the nineteenth century major changes relating to the investigation of death in the community occurred. In 1836, the first Births and Deaths Registration Act was passed, prompted by the public concern and panic caused by inaccurate 'parochial' recording of the actual numbers of deaths arising from epidemics such as cholera.

There was also growing concern that given the easy and uncontrolled access to numerous poisons, and inadequate medical investigation of the actual cause of death, many homicides were going undetected.

By then, the Coroner's fiscal responsibility had diminished and the Coroners Act of 1887 made significant changes here, repealing much of the earlier legislation. Coroners then became more concerned with determining the circumstances and the actual medical causes of sudden, violent and unnatural deaths for the benefit of the community as a whole.

DEATH CERTIFICATION

Section 22 of the Births and Deaths Registration Act 1953 provides that 'In the case of the death of any person who has been attended during his last illness by a registered medical practitioner, that practitioner shall sign a certificate in the prescribed form stating to the best of his knowledge and belief the cause of death and shall forthwith deliver that certificate to the registrar'.

Much unnecessary distress to grieving relatives waiting in a Register Office trying to register a death, and a great deal of subsequent anger directed at the individual doctor by those bereaved, can easily be avoided by taking care to ensure that the Medical Certificate of Cause of Death is completed properly and will not be rejected by the Registrar of Births and Deaths.

In the first instance this involves a knowledge and recognition of those deaths that must be reported to the coroner, as outlined below, in which case the Coroner's Office should be contacted by telephone for further guidance at the earliest possible opportunity prior to writing any certificate.

The Registrar of Births and Deaths scrutinises all Medical Certificates of Cause of Death, and has a statutory duty under section 41(1) of the Registration of Births and Deaths Regulations 1987 to report the death to the coroner if it is one:

'(a) in respect of which the deceased was not attended during his last illness by a registered medical practitioner; or

(b) in respect of which the registrar

(i) has been unable to obtain a duly completed certificate of the cause of death; or

    (ii) has received such a certificate with respect to which it appears to him, from the particulars contained in the certificate or otherwise, that the deceased was not seen by the certifying medical practitioner either after death or within 14 days before death; or

(c) the cause of which appears to be unknown; or

(d) which the registrar has reason to believe to have been unnatural or to have been caused by violence or neglect or by abortion, or to have been attended by suspicious circumstances; or

(e) which appears to the registrar to have occurred during an operation or before recovery from the effect of an anaesthetic; or

(f) which appears to the registrar from the contents of any medical certificate of cause of death to have been due to industrial disease or industrial poisoning.'[a]

Local arrangements usually exist for notifying deaths that occur within 24 hours of admission to hospital. This is not a statutory requirement, but the registrar may otherwise question a certificate if it appears that the patient may not have been in hospital long enough to enable the cause of death to be fully established, or if it appears that the patient was not attended during the last illness by a registered medical practitioner other than by hospital staff giving treatment in extremis.

Section 41(1) of the Registration of Births and Deaths Regulations defines most of the instances when a death must be reported to the coroner. It does not cover every case, however, an exception being deaths in custody which, rather than being notified through the registrar, will be reported directly to the coroner by the appropriate prison or police authority. The medical practitioner must be aware, though, that a prisoner who dies while a patient in hospital is still deemed legally to be in custody whether under guard or not, and such deaths whether natural or not must still be reported to the coroner rather than being registered in the normal manner.

Where the death is entirely natural and does not fall into any of the above categories, to ensure that the Medical Certificate of Cause of Death is acceptable to the Registrar of Births and Deaths, care must be taken to be certain that the certificate is completed correctly and the correct format employed. Useful advice on this was given in a letter to doctors from the Office of Population Censuses and Surveys in 1990.[b]

This reminded doctors that the certificates served both legal and statistical purposes, and pointed out some of the common errors in certification that occur. It specifically mentions that there is no need to record the mode of dying, as this does not assist in deriving mortality statistics, and stresses that it is even more important not to complete a certificate where the mode of dying, for example shock, uraemia or asphyxia, is the only entry.

It emphasises the need to avoid the use of abbreviations at all times. This can clearly be a source of ambiguity and confusion, particularly where abbreviations are shared, such as 'MI' which might mean mitral incompetence or myocardial infarction, or 'MS' which might mean mitral stenosis or multiple sclerosis.

Where the fatal disease process is one that is often recognised to be employment-related but is known not to be in that particular patient, then the addition of the words 'non-industrial' on the certificate after the cause of death can avoid subsequent enquiry by the registrar.

It is also worth observing that there are very useful notes and directions accompanying books of blank Medical Certificates of Cause of Death.[c] Following these will avoid many of the common problems that arise, for example relating to the correct inclusion and positioning of any relevant antecedent diseases or conditions, and will ensure that part I, and where appropriate part II, are filled in correctly and in a logical sequence.

Problems leading to the rejection of certificates frequently arise when junior doctors, uncertain of the exact cause of death or what they should write, are asked to complete the Medical Certificate of Cause of Death. If in any doubt they should always consult their senior colleagues in these circumstances. A survey published in 1993, however, revealed similar and significant numbers of failures to recognise which deaths are reportable across all grades of doctor from junior to senior.[d]

Any doctor who is uncertain, therefore, regardless of seniority, would be best advised to seek the guidance of the local Coroner's Office to resolve any doubts and to avoid any subsequent problems and distress to relatives.

Problems can also arise from a doctor's desire (albeit well-intentioned) to keep certain sensitive diagnoses off the Medical Certificate of Cause of Death, and this has been discussed in the chapter on confidentiality (see Ch. 6).

Aspects of transplantation have also been discussed elsewhere in this book, but it is worthy of note that, in addition to the normal requirements relating to consent that must be satisfied prior to any transplant, by section 1(5) of the Human Tissue Act 1961, the consent of the coroner must also be obtained prior to any transplant 'where a person has reason to believe that an inquest may be required to be held on any body or that a post-mortem examination of any body may be required by the coroner'.

At the present time, about a third of all deaths in England and Wales are reported to coroners. In 1994, out of a total of 551 600 deaths, 185 000 were reported, and the outcome of these deaths will now be examined.

Natural deaths

In those circumstances where further enquiry indicates that a reported death is due to natural causes and does not require a post mortem examination, the coroner will issue a Form 100A, which notifies the registrar that the death was due to natural causes, and the attending doctor will be advised to complete a Medical Certificate of the Cause of Death in the usual manner.

In the majority of cases reported to coroners, however, a post mortem examination is still required to ascertain the cause of death, although the proportion of cases requiring this has been declining slowly over the years. If the cause of death is found to be natural at autopsy, the coroner will issue a Form 100B, which notifies the registrar of the cause of death, and that no further action is to be taken.

Upon receipt of either the Medical Certificate of the Cause of Death from the attending doctor, or Form 100B from the coroner, the registrar is able to register the death and issue a disposal certificate to allow for arrangements to be made to dispose of the body.

In 1994, post mortem examinations were ordered on 125 200 of the 185 000 reported deaths. This proportion has declined steadily as the number of deaths requiring neither post mortem nor inquest has increased.

Unnatural deaths and inquests

In cases where the cause of death is found not to be natural, the coroner has a statutory duty to conduct an inquest under Section 8(1) of the Coroners Act 1988, which provides that:

'Where a coroner is informed that a body of a person ("the deceased") is lying within his district and there is reasonable cause to suspect that the deceased

    (a) has died a violent or unnatural death;

(b) has died a sudden death of which the cause is unknown; or
(c) has died in prison, or in such a place or in such circumstances as to require an inquest under any other Act,

then, whether the cause of death arose within his district or not, the coroner shall as soon as practicable hold an inquest into the death of the deceased either with or, subject to subsection (3), without a jury.'

Prior to 1926, every inquest had to be held with a jury, but nowadays, in the majority of inquests, the coroner sits alone. Section 8(3) of the Coroners Act 1988 provides that:

'If it appears to a coroner, either before he proceeds to hold an inquest or in the course of an inquest begun without a jury, that there is reason to suspect

(a) that the death occurred in prison or in such a place or in such circumstances as to require an inquest under any other Act;
(b) that the death occurred while the deceased was in police custody, or resulted from an injury caused by a police officer in the purported execution of his duty;
(c) that the death was caused by an accident, poisoning or disease notice of which is required to be given under any Act to a government department, to any inspector or other officer of a government department or to an inspector appointed under section 19 of the Health and Safety at Work etc. Act 1974; or
(d) that the death occurred in circumstances the continuance or possible recurrence of which is prejudicial to the health or safety of the public or any section of the public,

he shall proceed to summon a jury in the manner required by subsection (2).'

The conduct of an inquest is governed by The Coroners Rules 1984, and the function and ambit of an inquest was usefully examined and clearly re-affirmed by the Court of Appeal in *R* v *North Humberside Coroner, ex parte Jamieson* **[1994]**.[1]

Rule 36 (Matters to be Ascertained at Inquest) provides that:

'(1) The proceedings and evidence at inquest shall be directed solely to ascertaining the following matters, namely
    (a) who the deceased was;
    (b) how, when and where the deceased came by his death;
    (c) the particulars for the time being required by the Registration Acts to be registered concerning the death.
(2) Neither the coroner nor the jury shall express any opinion on any other matters.'

Rule 42 (Verdict) provides that:

'No verdict shall be framed in such a way as to appear to determine any question of

---

1 *R* v *North Humberside Coroner, ex parte Jamieson* [1994] 3 WLR 82 CA

(a) criminal liability on the part of a named person, or
(b) civil liability.'

It is important to appreciate that an inquest is a fact finding enquiry rather than a fault finding trial, and the proceedings are inquisitorial rather than adversarial in nature but, as the Master of the Rolls indicated giving the judgment of the court in *R* v *North Humberside Coroner, ex parte Jamieson*, it is the duty of the coroner to 'ensure that the relevant facts were fully, fairly and fearlessly investigated'.

The coroner will initially examine a witness on oath, after which relevant questions may be put to the witness by any of those with a proper interest in the proceedings, either in person or by counsel or solicitor. Those people who have this entitlement to examine witnesses are defined in Rule 20 of the Coroners Rules.

Evidence given on oath before a coroner may subsequently be used in proceedings in other courts. Rule 22 provides that:

(1) no witness at an inquest shall be obliged to answer any question tending to incriminate himself, and
(2) where it appears to the coroner that a witness has been asked such a question, the coroner shall inform the witness that he may refuse to answer.

This privilege does not allow a witness to refuse to enter the witness box, and the protection against self-incrimination that it offers applies only to criminal offences, and not to possible civil or disciplinary proceedings.

If a doctor feels that his or her professional conduct may be called into question, then this should be discussed with the relevant defence organisation in good time, so that the possible need for the doctor to be legally represented can be addressed.

Inquests were held on 20 800, or about 11%, of deaths reported to coroners in 1994. The commonest verdicts were death by accident or misadventure, which was recorded in 47% of cases that year, and suicide, recorded in 18%. The Home Office Statistics of Deaths Reported to Coroners in 1994 also reveal that the verdicts of death from industrial diseases almost doubled in 10 years from 5% in 1984 to 9% in 1994, and that verdicts of death from drug abuse have also increased.[e]

Treasure trove

Apart from those duties relating to unnatural death that are provided by s.8(1) of the Coroners Act 1988, one last vestige of the coroner's medieval duties remains. Section 30 of the Coroners Act 1988 provides that a coroner shall continue to have jurisdiction to inquire into any treasure which is found in his district, although in modern times this has more to do with the preservation of antiquities rather than for any financial benefit to the Crown.

REFERENCES

a Registration of Births and Deaths Regulations 1987
b Office of Population Censuses and Surveys 1990 Completion of Medical Certificates of Cause of Death (letter to doctors). Office of Population Censuses and Surveys, London
c Notes and directions accompanying books of blank Medical Certificates of Cause of Death
d Start R D, Delargy-Aziz Y, Dorries C P, Silocks P B, Cotton D W K 1993 Clinicians and the coronial system: ability of clinicians to recognise reportable deaths. British Medical Journal 306: 1038–1041
e Home Office 1995 Statistics of deaths reported to coroners: England and Wales 1994. Home Office Statistical Bulletin 6/95. Home Office, London

FURTHER READING

Health Departments of Great Britain and Northern Ireland Working Party 1983 Cadaveric organs for transplantation; a code of practice including the diagnosis of brain death. Department of Health, London
Hunnisett R F 1961 The medieval coroner. Cambridge University Press, Cambridge
Matthews P, Foreman J (eds) 1993 Jervis on coroners, 11th edn. Sweet & Maxwell, London

8. Living wills

Diana Tribe, Gill Korgaonkar

INTRODUCTION

A living will is usually a written document which is designed to give doctors advance instructions about treatment preferences in the event of the 'declarant' suffering mental incapacity and/or terminal illness. It can also contain instructions about the appointment of a healthcare proxy who would have the right to be consulted, have the authority to make decisions and represent the declarant's views in the event of incompetency.

The 'living will' (so called because it will take effect in the person's lifetime, unlike a traditional will concerned with distribution of the testator's property which takes effect only on death) could give instructions that, in the event of the declarant suffering a terminal illness, permanent unconsciousness or persistent vegetative state (PVS), life-sustaining or life-prolonging treatment be withheld or withdrawn. Conversely, the declarant could make a 'life prolonging declaration'[a] outlining the circumstances in which he wished to be kept alive for as long as reasonably possible.

The legal status of such documents has been the subject of much recent debate, both in the United Kingdom and in the United States. Their validity has not been tested in the English courts, although recent case law[1,2] indicates that they are almost certainly enforceable at common law. The Law Commission has, however, recommended that legislation should be passed which would give statutory recognition to 'anticipated decisions' which would bind doctors.[b] It further recommends that a person should have the right to appoint a 'medical treatment attorney' to make treatment decisions on that person's behalf on incompetency.

---

1 *Airedale NHS Trust v Bland* [1993] 1 All ER 821; [1993] HL 2 WLR 317. Tony Bland was severaly brain-damaged in the Hillsborough Stadium disaster in 1989 and existed in a persistent vegetative state until the House of Lords allowed him to die in 1993

2 *Re T (Adult: Refusal of Medical Treatment)* [1992] 4 All ER 649

Background

The introduction of a living will was first proposed in the USA by Luis Kutner at a Euthanasia Society of America meeting in 1967. The first statutory support came in California's Natural Death Act 1976. Since then 'hybrid statutes' have become common which allow both the making of a living will and the appointment of a healthcare proxy; these have become known as 'advance directives'. Some 40 States have made statutory provision for their adoption and it is estimated that approximately 9% of Americans have executed some form of 'advance directive' stipulating how they wish medical treatment decisions to be handled in the event of their becoming incompetent.[c]

In the UK the Voluntary Euthanasia Society has made available living wills since the early 1970s. They have also been championed since the mid-1980s by Age Concern, which, in conjunction with the Centre of Medical Law and Ethics, produced a working party report on 'The living will: consent to treatment at the end of life'[d] The Terence Higgins Trust produced a living will form in 1992 which is designed to take effect when the declarant becomes 'unable to communicate and cannot take part in decisions about my medical care.'[e]

In November 1992 the British Medical Association (BMA) published a statement on advance directives which strongly supports them in principle, as it sees them as giving 'significant benefits . . . within the framework of continuing doctor-patient dialogue'. It is not, however, in favour of their being legally binding although it accepts that doctors will normally comply with their contents. It recognises, however, that doctors who have a conscientious objection to curtailing treatment should have the right to transfer that patient's care to another practitioner.[f]

THE COMMON LAW RULES ON CONSENT TO TREATMENT

The underpinning philosophy of the living will, to which the law gives effect, is the individual's right to self-determination. This legal right is encapsulated in the now famous statement of Justice Cardozo. 'Every human being of adult years and sound mind has a right to determine what shall be done with his own body'.[3] Self-

---

3 *Schloendorff* v *Society of New York Hospitals* 211 NY 128, 105 NE 93 [1914]

determination clearly encompasses the right to refuse medical treatment. This has been echoed recently in an English case where Lord Donaldson said, in relation to a mentally competent person's right to grant or withhold consent to medical treatment, 'This right of choice is not limited to decisions which others might regard as sensible. It exists notwithstanding that the reasons for making the choice are rational, irrational, unknown or even non-existent'.[2] Thus, for a doctor who undertakes any treatment without the express or implied consent of the competent patient,[g] even if the treatment is perceived to be in that patient's 'best interests', the doctor will be acting unlawfully and will be liable in damages to that patient in the tort of battery and/or negligence.[4,5] Criminal liability might also ensue.[h] Life-saving treatment administered in an emergency where it is impossible to obtain consent because the patient is unconscious (for example following a road traffic accident) will not incur liability, either on the juridical basis that the patient has 'impliedly' consented[6] or on the basis of the doctrine of 'necessity'[7] (i.e. that the doctor was acting in the patient's best interest). The exception to this basic rule is where the patient has clearly indicated in advance that consent in such circumstances would be withheld. Thus, in *Malette* v *Shulman*[8] where a blood transfusion was given to an unconscious card-carrying Jehovah's Witness on the grounds that it was in the patient's 'best interests', the patient's right to self-determination was upheld and damages granted. It would therefore follow that if a person had made a living will indicating that they wished to withhold consent in certain stipulated circumstances, a doctor who sought to disregard such an instruction would incur legal liability.[i]

Where a person has never been competent to consent to treatment the defence of necessity will again avail the doctor where medical treatment is administered in the 'best interests'[j] of that patient. Indeed, a failure to treat in such circumstances could give rise to liability. If a doctor makes a decision that it would be in the 'best interests' of an adult patient to receive 'non-therapeutic' treatment (for example, a sterilization), the High Court alone has an

---

4 See, for example, *Chatterton* v *Gerson* [1981] 1 All ER 257
5 *Sidaway* v *Board of Governors of the Bethlem Royal Hospital and the Maudsley Hospital* [1985] AC 871
6 *Mohr* v *Williams* [1905] 104 NW 12 (Sup Ct Min)
7 *Re F (a mental patient: sterilization)* [1990] 2 AC 1
8 *Malette* v *Shulman* [1990] 67 DLR (4th) 321 (Ont CA)

exclusive right to grant or withhold consent to such treatment in the patient's 'best interests'.[7]

The same rule would apply to a situation where the patient was originally competent but, because of illness or accident, is no longer so, in the absence of his having made a legally binding anticipatory choice. In *Bland*[1] (see also Ch. 4) the English courts were faced with two important questions. Firstly, whether artificial feeding constituted 'medical treatment' and secondly, if it did, whether this 'medical treatment' could be withheld from a patient in a persistent vegetative state[k] in circumstances where it would inevitably cause his death. Both these questions were answered in the affirmative. The judges in the House of Lords agreed that sanctity of life was a fundamental principle of law but all agreed that it was not an absolute one. There is, they said, no absolute legal rule that a patient's life must be prolonged by medical treatment, regardless of the circumstances. Thus the law does not authorise the forcible feeding of patients on hunger strike, nor the temporary keeping alive of terminally ill patients, where to do so would merely prolong their suffering. Where treatment has no 'therapeutic value' and there is no prospect of an improvement in the patient's condition, 'the futility of the treatment justifies its termination' (per Lord Goff). The court also made it clear that where people indicate in advance that they do not want life-sustaining treatment in the event of their falling into a state which they themselves conceive of as being intolerable, 'the right of self-determination entails that such wishes should be respected'.[1] They also made it clear that in such situations the High Court has the exclusive right to grant consent to the withholding of treatment. Whilst the views of the relatives were accorded weight by the courts, it is clear that relatives of incapacitated patients do not have legal capacity to grant or withhold consent on an adult incompetent's behalf in the absence of their having validly executed a healthcare proxy form:

'There seems to be a view in the legal profession that in . . . emergency circumstances the next of kin should be asked to consent on behalf of the patient and that, if possible, treatment should be postponed until that consent has been obtained. This is a misconception because the next of kin has no legal right either to consent or to refuse consent. This is not to say that it is an undesirable practice if the interests of the patient will not be adversely affected by any consequential delay. I say this because contact with the next of kin may reveal that the patient has made an anticipatory choice which, if clearly established and if applicable in the circumstances—two major "ifs"—would bind the practitioner . . .'.[m]

LIVING WILL FORMS

For an anticipatory refusal of medical treatment to be effective at common law it must meet four important criteria.[2] Firstly, the patient must be competent at the time of refusal (that is, *inter alia*, that he must be free from the influence of drugs, or not be suffering from mental illness). Secondly, his free will must not have been overborne by the influence of a third party; thirdly, he must have understood in broad terms the nature and effect of the treatment which is being refused (or consented to); and finally the refusal must cover the actual situation in which the treatment is needed.

This fourth criterion may allow the courts (and doctors) the ability to 'undermine the law's apparent commitment to a patient's right to self-determination.'[n] If a living will is not drafted in other than general terms it might be comparatively easy to argue that it was not intended to apply in the circumstances which subsequently arise. There is evidence from the USA that many living wills fail to give sufficiently clear instructions and thus the medical profession feel uncertain about applying them.[o] For example, Florida's living will directs that when a person is in a terminal condition 'life-prolonging procedures be withheld or withdrawn when the application of such procedures would serve only to prolong artificially the process of dying'. Can it, for example, be inferred that the declarant categorically wishes to forgo cardiopulmonary resuscitation (CPR)? Indeed research evidence from the USA suggests that, of those people who had made a living will, over one third had not communicated this fact to their doctor, nor had they specifically discussed their CPR preferences.[p] Furthermore, research in the UK indicates that 'patients who are acutely unwell may make decisions that are influenced by their condition at this point in time and it is important to recognise that these decisions may not be maintained'.[q] Because living wills are usually made when illness is but an abstract concept to the declarant, it is clearly important to appreciate that that person's views may subsequently change.

The Terence Higgins Trust living will form recommends that intending declarants discuss it with a doctor (though such people are under no obligation to do so) and, if this is done, the form provides space for the name and address of that doctor to be included. It allows for a declarant to give instructions about both general and particular forms of medical treatment and to have his wishes temporarily disregarded whilst a named person/s is given the opportunity to make contact with the declarant. A healthcare proxy may also be appointed and the will has to be signed by a person over the age of 18 who is not the spouse or partner, relative, potential beneficiary or appointed healthcare proxy of the declarant or the spouse or partner of any of these individuals.

As previously noted, the legal validity of such a will has not yet been tested in the English courts. It is assumed, on the basis of the law outlined above, that it will be legally binding and thus a doctor who acts in contravention of its provisions will be liable both in tort and under the criminal law. There may be a defence if it can be argued that the will has not been sufficiently clearly drafted to cover the eventuality or that there is evidence that the declarant has since changed his mind.

The remaining problem, which again the courts have not as yet been required to address, is whether the effectiveness of a living will could cease by mere passage of time. An extended time period between the making of the living will and the onset of the relevant incapacity may give rise to doubts as to whether the declarant's wishes have changed in the intervening period. The BMA recommended[r] that they be revised every five years but there is no reason to believe that the English common law would make a presumption of automatic revocation after any given period of time.[s]

The right of children to make living wills

There is no indication on the Terence Higgins Trust's living will form that the declarant should be over the age of 18. The Family Law Reform Act 1969[t] provides that a person aged 16 years and over may give a valid consent to medical treatment. Furthermore, the House of Lords has made it clear[9] that a person who is under the age of 16 years who is of sufficient understanding and intelligence is also capable of giving valid consent in English law. The question arises as to whether a person under the age of 18 has a comparable right to *refuse* treatment, particularly in circumstances where this will inevitably lead to death. In two important cases[10,11] the Court of Appeal held that a minor's right to refuse medical treatment was not synonymous with his right to consent to such treatment. Whilst it accepted that a minor child below the age of 16 has the right to consent to treatment 'when the child achieves a

---

9 *Gillick* v *West Norfolk and Wisbech Area Health Authority* [1986] AC 112
10 *Re R (a minor) (wardship: medical treatment)* [1991] 4 All ER 177, and
11 *Re W (a minor) (medical treatment)* [1992] 4 All ER 627

sufficient understanding and intelligence to enable him or her to understand fully what is proposed'[u] and that such consent could not be challenged by the parents (or others with parental responsibility), the judges accepted that the *refusal* of consent by the competent child (under the age of *18 years*) could be overridden by parents or the courts.

Thus a minor's capacity to make a valid living will stipulating the circumstances in which he wished to have life saving treatment withheld is doubtful. However, when Tony Bland went to support Liverpool in the football match against Nottingham Forest at Hillsborough he was only 17 years of age. The court judgment seems to accept, albeit implicitly, that a minor's declaration about future medical treatment in such circumstances would be legally recognised.[1] There was, however, a parental wish that his treatment be discontinued in this case.

It is also questionable whether a pregnant woman can effectively refuse consent to life saving treatment at common law if this treatment is in the interests of both patient and fetus.[12] This would suggest, therefore, that the effectiveness of a living will would be suspended during pregnancy (see below).

THE LAW COMMISSION'S PROPOSALS

The Law Commission has made the following important proposals:[v]

1. Legislation should provide for the scope and effect of anticipatory decisions.
2. If a patient is incapacitated (subject to the caveats discussed below) a clearly established anticipatory decision should be as effective as the contemporaneous decision of the patient would be in the circumstances to which it is applicable.
3. There should be a rebuttable presumption that an anticipatory decision is clearly established if it is in writing, signed by the maker (with appropriate provision for signing at his direction), and witnessed by (one) person who is not the maker's medical treatment attorney.
4. An anticipatory decision should be regarded as ineffective to the extent that it purports to refuse pain relief or 'basic care', including nursing care and spoon-feeding.

---

12 *Re S (Adult: Refusal of medical treatment)* [1992] 4 All ER 671

5. An anticipatory decision may be revoked orally or in writing at any time when the maker has the capacity to do so. There should be no automatic revocation after a period of time.

6. A treatment provider who acts in accordance with an apparently valid and continuing anticipatory decision should only be liable to any civil or criminal proceedings if he or she does so in bad faith or without reasonable care.

7. It should be an offence to falsify or forge an advance directive; or to conceal, alter or destroy a directive without the authority of its maker. These offences should apply to a written revocation of an advance directive as they do to the directive itself.

It is important to note that the Law Commission did not think it appropriate to recommend that a living will should cease to be effective in pregnancy.

If and when these proposals will become law is, as yet, uncertain.

CONCLUSION

It has been argued that a living will is a 'white, middle-class approach to life planning which is at odds with how many people actually lead their lives, and may not even be the standard for that class.'[w] Clearly, however, living wills provide an important mechanism for involving people in decisions about their medical care which has become increasingly relevant as medical science has progressed.

REFERENCES

a   See, for example, the 'Life-prolonging procedures declaration' in the State of Indiana's Living Wills and Life Prolonging Procedures Act 1985

b   Law Commission 1993 Consultation Paper 129: Mentally incapacitated adults and decision making: medical treatment and research. Law Commission, London

c   Gelfand G 1987 Living will statutes: the first decade. Wisconsin Law Review 737

d   Lush D 1993 Advance directives and living wills. Journal of the Royal College of Physicians of London 27:3:274

e   Copies of the Living Will form are available from the Terence Higgins Trust, 52–54 Grays Inn Road, London WC1X 8JU, UK. Telephone: 0171 405 2381

f   British Medical Association 1992 Statement of advance directives. British Medical Association, London

g   A competent person may be defined as an individual who is able to understand and appreciate the nature and consequences of a decision to accept or refuse treatment

h   Battery is also a crime both at common law and under the Offences Against the Person Act 1861 (ss18, 20 and 45)

i   Legal problems, of course, might arise in regard to, *inter alia*, the construction of
    the words used in the 'will' and whether they covered the eventuality, whether
    there was any indication that the declarant had changed his mind between the
    making of the 'will' and the eventuality, and in respect of his capacity in the first
    place to make a valid 'will'
j   The 'best interests' test is sometimes described as an objective test and requires
    the doctor to provide the treatment that would be most 'beneficial to the patient'
k   A patient in a PVS was defined in the American case *Re Quinlan* [1976] 70 NJ 10
    as a person who 'remains with the capacity to maintain the vegetative parts of
    the neurological function but who no longer has any cognitive function'
l   Per Lord Justice Hoffman
m   Lord Donaldson, Master of the Rolls in *Re T* (see case 2)
n   Kennedy I, Grubb A 1995 Medical law, text with materials, 2nd edn.
    Butterworths, London
o   Walker R M, Schonwetter R S, Kramer D R, Robinson B E 1995 Living wills
    and resuscitation preferences in an elderly population. Archives of Internal
    Medicine: 155
p   ibid
q   Potter J M, Stewart D, Duncan G 1994 Living wills: would sick people change
    their minds? Postgraduate Medical Journal 70:818
r   British Medical Association 1992 Statement of advance directives. British
    Medical Association, London
s   See Law Commission 1993 Consultation Paper 129: Mentally incapacitated
    adults and decision-making: medical treatment and research. Law Commission,
    London
t   s8(1)
u   per Lord Scarman in *Gillick* at p 423
v   Law Commission 1993 Consultation Paper 129, as in note s above
w   King P 1991 The authority of families to make medical decisions for
    incompetent patients after the *Cruzan* decision. Law, Medicine and Health Care
    19:76

9. Euthanasia

Diana Brahams

INTRODUCTION

Euthanasia is defined in Butterworths Medical Dictionary (2nd edn) as '1. The process of dying easily, quietly and painlessly. 2. The act or practice of procuring, as an act of mercy, the easy and painless death of a patient who has an incurable and intractably painful and distressing disease.'

It is the second of these two definitions of euthanasia, namely the carrying out of a deliberate act with the primary aim of bringing the patient's life to an end whether or not the patient agrees or requests it, albeit as an act of mercy, which may expose the doctor to a criminal prosecution for murder or attempted murder in the UK. In Holland, by contrast, while voluntary euthanasia — i.e. with the agreement of the patient — remains a crime, no prosecution will be brought if certain specified criteria are complied with by the doctors concerned.[a] However, evidence suggests that attitudes have become considerably more relaxed and that many more deaths result from pro-actively achieved euthanasia than appear on the official records.

UK legal issues

In the UK, the legality of the doctor's conduct will depend on his intentions and his objectives. If the doctor's *primary* objective was to relieve serious pain and suffering with the incidental consequence that the patient's life was shortened and indeed death resulted quite rapidly, this may be lawfully induced euthanasia, namely, a painless and easy death. This is sometimes known as the doctrine of 'double effect' and is well illustrated by Lord Devlin's direction to the jury in the case of *R* v *Bodkin Adams*.[1] Conversely, if the doctor's primary intention was to bring life to an end —

---

1 *R* v *Bodkin Adams* [1957] CLR 365

albeit to prevent further suffering — e.g. by the administration of a lethal substance with no known analgesic indications such as potassium chloride, then the patient might achieve an easy and painless death but the doctor (or any other perpetrator) risks a charge of murder or attempted murder if his conduct is investigated. The prosecution case *inter alia* in the Bodkin Adams trial was that the doctor was an unprincipled, greedy man, who murdered an elderly patient, Mrs Morrell, in 1950 by prescribing and/or giving her fatally large doses of morphine and heroin in order to accelerate the receipt of a legacy she had provided for him in her will. There were rumours that this was a pattern of behaviour regularly repeated among his large elderly clientele, though this evidence could not be adduced at the trial of the Morrell case. Dr Bodkin Adams' motives were therefore attacked and thereby also his intent in giving fatally large quantities of drugs in the circumstances. Further, when questioned initially by the police some 6 years on, Dr Bodkin Adams astonishingly and almost certainly untruthfully made the damaging admission that he had injected nearly all the drugs which he had prescribed (which were massive and would have been fatal to the patient).

In Lord Devlin's review of this celebrated trial over which he had presided so many years before, he said:

In the Adams case the [Gordian] knot was in the beginning formed — as the tangles in the legal process which lead to injustice so often are — out of the lie told by the accused when he said that he had himself injected all that he had prescribed. I do not doubt, first, that he made this statement; second, that it was untrue.[b]

However, it was Lord Devlin's famous direction to the jury on the law relating to easing the passing by doctors, which he goes on to quote in his review and which explains the basic English legal position succinctly.[c]

Murder is the cutting short of life, whether by years, months or weeks. It does not matter that Mrs Morrell's days were numbered. '. . . But that does not mean that a doctor who is aiding the sick and the dying has to calculate in minutes or even hours, and perhaps not in days and weeks, the effect upon a patient's life of the medicines which he administers or else be in peril of a charge of murder. If the first purpose of medicine, the restoration of health, can no longer be achieved, there is still much for a doctor to do, and he is entitled to do all that is proper and necessary to relieve pain and suffering, even if the measures he takes may incidentally shorten life . . .'. This is not because there is a special defence for medical men but because no act is murder which does not cause death. We are not dealing here with the philosophical or technical cause, but with the commonsense cause. The cause of death is the illness or the injury, '. . . and the proper medical treatment that is administered and that has an incidental effect on determining the exact moment of death is not the cause of death in any sensible use of the term. But . . . no doctor, nor any man, no more in the case of the dying than of the healthy, has the right deliberately to cut the thread of life . . .'

It was not contended by the defence that Dr Adams had any right to make any determination.

Lord Devlin told the jury that details of the course of the illness which preceded the vital period in November 1950 were 'inessentials'.

'Not a pretty story: lavish use of heroin, angling for a legacy, being taken out of the will and put back again, the cremation form which you may think is false.' But there is a big difference between this and murder. Even if they thought the doctor a fraudulent rogue, 'fraud and murder are poles apart.'[d]

In all, the summing up was favourable to the defence. After 46 minutes' deliberation, the jury returned a verdict of not guilty. Dr Adams had already been committed for trial on another indictment in respect of another patient, to which the Attorney-General entered a 'nolle prosequi' which Devlin considered was an abuse of process by the Prosecution to prevent a verdict of acquittal. However, the fact was that so far as the wider world was concerned, the Prosecution had been defeated on one indictment and had thrown in his hand on the other!

The general principles then are reasonably clear. However, the application to individual cases may give rise not only to legal difficulties but also to philosophical ones, and the question arises whether a doctor who intends to end a patient's life as an act of mercy should automatically be liable to a conviction for murder or at the least of attempted murder. Should it depend on whether or not the doctor is acting in response to a direct request from the patient, given that the patient is able to communicate his wishes? Should aiding and abetting a suicide in such circumstances remain a crime even though suicide itself has not been a crime since the Suicide Act 1961 was passed? A more pragmatic approach is taken in Holland, namely, the agreement not to prosecute in what are deemed to be appropriate circumstances. This however leaves doctors vulnerable and patients open to abuses of the system. Thus the 'thin end of the wedge' argument is at the root of most of the opposition to the legalisation of 'mercy killing' in almost any circumstances (save perhaps the killing of a dying prisoner of war where torture and death at the hands of the enemy are inevitable).

Following the recent cases of *R* v *Cox*[2] and *Airedale NHS Trust* v *Bland*[3] (see below), a committee set up by the House of Lords considered the legal and ethical issues arising from the problems raised by the care of the dying which were exacerbated by technological aids to prolong life, arguably achieving no useful purpose. The Lords committee strongly endorsed the right of the patient to refuse consent to medical treatment, and for the better regulation of treatment to avoid, where possible, the commencement of treatment in cases with hopeless prognoses, but rejected the calls for a change in the law to legalise voluntary euthanasia.

The Committee considered both the views of those who advocate voluntary euthanasia and those whose experiences of deaths were neither peaceful nor uplifting. It concluded:

Ultimately, however, we do not believe these arguments are sufficient reason to weaken society's prohibition of intentional killing. That prohibition is the cornerstone of the law and of social relationships. It protects each one of us impartially, embodying the belief that all are equal. We do not wish that protection to be diminished and we therefore recommend that there should be no change in the law to permit euthanasia. One reason for this conclusion is that we do not think it possible to set secure limits on voluntary euthanasia . . . to create an exception to the general prohibition of intentional killing would inevitably open the way to its further erosion whether by design, by inadvertence, or by the human tendency to test the limits of any regulation.[e]

The Committee then went on to consider the law of double effect — the *Bodkin Adams* rationale:

In the small and diminishing number of cases in which pain and distress cannot be satisfactorily controlled, we are satisfied that the professional judgment of the health-care team can be exercised to enable increasing doses of medication (whether analgesics or sedatives) to be given in order to provide relief, even if this shortens life . . . we have confidence in the ability of the medical profession to discern when the administration of drugs has been inappropriate or excessive. An additional safeguard is that increased emphasis on team working makes it improbable that doctors could deliberately and recklessly shorten the lives of their patients without their actions arousing suspicion.[f]

A doctor's motives and 'intent'

Thus it is that in the UK, acts taken by doctors with the primary intent to end life will be unlawful and may end with a conviction

2 *R* v *Cox* 1992 1238 Crown
3 *Airedale NHS Trust* v *Bland* (HL) 1993 2 WLR 317

for attempted murder or murder itself, if death can be proved to have resulted from the doctor's action rather than the underlying condition. English law does not recognise a separate category of 'mercy killing', and the doctor's motives (his reasons for acting may be altruistic and driven by compassion) must be separated from what his legal 'intent' was when carrying out his actions. Obviously, the motives of the doctor may shed light on what was his legal 'intent' and, if he is convicted (depending on whether he is a potential re-offender and a danger to the public), motives such as altruism and compassion, in contrast to financial reward resulting from the patient's death, may be taken into account by the judge in deciding on an appropriate sentence. However, if the doctor is convicted of murder, there will be no opportunity for judicial discretion as murder still carries a mandatory life sentence[g] (though there can be an early release on licence).

In the highly publicised case of *R* v *Cox*, which was considered by the House of Lords Committee, Dr Nigel Cox, a consultant physician, administered a lethal injection of potassium chloride to relieve the patient's unbearable suffering in the terminal stages of her illness. The injection was recorded in the patient's notes. At all times, Dr Cox enjoyed the full confidence of the patient and her family. However, Dr Cox's choice of potassium chloride was questioned, as it is a substance with no analgesic qualities (save that it causes death and thereby can be said to end suffering) and thus deprived him of the defence of double effect, thereby putting him outside the protection of the law. Had he instead opted for a large dose of morphine which had resulted in the patient's death, he would almost certainly not have been prosecuted for attempted murder, and if he had been, it is virtually certain that he would have been acquitted.[h]

Dr Cox (like Dr Bodkin Adams) never stepped into the witness box to testify and thus avoided being subjected to any cross-examination by the Prosecution. The jury were reluctant but were nonetheless left with no option but to find him guilty of intending the attempted murder of his patient owing to his administration of potassium chloride. Dr Cox was sentenced to 12 months in prison suspended for 1 year. However, following an inquiry by the health authority, he was promptly reinstated in his post as a consultant physician (subject to a limited period of supervision and restrictions on some aspects of practice).

Causation

Dr Cox was not charged with murder but with attempted murder, and this was due to potential difficulties in proving causation because the patient had already been cremated by the time a nurse who read the notes had alerted the hospital manager and police inquiries were instigated. Certainly, with no body for the forensic pathologists to review, there could have been technical evidential difficulties in proving that it was the potassium chloride rather than the overwhelming and terminal illness that had caused the death — though reportedly, the patient died very quickly after the potassium chloride was injected.

Further, the prosecution would have been mindful of the earlier case of Dr Stephen Lodwig, a junior hospital doctor, who in 1989 was accused of murdering a terminally ill cancer patient suffering from unbearable pain by administering a lethal injection comprising a combination of potassium chloride and lignocaine.[4] On 15 March 1990, the prosecution decided to offer no evidence at an Old Bailey hearing and Dr Lodwig was formally cleared of all charges. In 1981, in R v Arthur[5] the Prosecution was criticised by the trial judge as the evidence on causation foundered. Dr Leonard Arthur was a paediatrician accused of the murder of a very sick neonate suffering from Down's syndrome by ordering the administration of a regimen allowing for 'nursing care only' and the administration of substantial doses of dihydrocodeine and water. The charge of murder had to be abandoned during the trial and reduced to one of attempted murder.[i] His motives were considered unimpeachable and his practices said to be in accordance with a responsible body of paediatric opinion, and Dr Arthur was acquitted. However, Dr Arthur's decision to allow the baby to die seems to have been made on the basis that he was a Down's syndrome baby and his parents 'did not want it to survive' and not because he considered the prognosis necessarily hopeless. This appears to be in conflict with the earlier Court of Appeal decision in Re B (a Minor)[6] and subsequent decisions.[j]

A jury's reluctance to convict an honest, caring doctor in these circumstances is understandable and manifest. However, even where there may be a question mark over the doctor's motives as well as his legal intent, juries may well feel unhappy about convict-

4 R v Lodwig [1990] Lancet 335: 718
5 R v Arthur [1981] 12(1) Crown Court
6 Re B (a Minor) [1981] 1 WLR 1421

ing him of homicide or attempted homicide, particularly if the patient's family is supportive of the doctor's actions.

The defence of double effect which was successfully argued on behalf of Dr Bodkin Adams was also employed in the defence of Dr Arthur. Neither Bodkin Adams nor Arthur testified and both were acquitted of homicide or attempted homicide.

In Arthur's case there were positive steps which the Prosecution alleged were deliberately taken with a view to causing the baby's death, namely prescribing dihydrocodeine in substantial quantity, combined with negative steps, namely the failure to feed the baby with anything more sustaining than water and dihydrocodeine. The Defence case was that the baby had legitimately and humanely been 'allowed to die'. The baby's condition was innately so poor that it could not be proved that Dr Arthur's regimen had caused its early death, hence the reduction of the charge during the trial to one of attempted murder.

Though Mr Justice Ognall, the trial judge in *R* v *Cox* has since indicated he believed the official decision to prosecute Dr Cox for attempted murder rather than for murder to have been a pragmatic Prosecution decision, no jury, he believed, would be so unwilling to convict a well motivated consultant physician of murder when his aim had been to relieve terrible suffering in a terminally ill, elderly patient. Accordingly, a charge of attempted murder was more likely to result in a conviction by the jury![k]

Such cases where there have been positive interventionist steps taken by the doctor which affect life expectancy and outcome should be distinguished again from cases where the patient has a hopeless prognosis, and medical treatment, which may include intravenous hydration and nutrition, is not considered to be achieving any benefit for the patient and thus is not in the patient's best interests. In such cases when medical treatment is discontinued or in some cases not started at all, and death follows, this is lawful. It may well not achieve euthanasia under Definition 1 (see above, Introduction) and may be an apparently cruel and protracted process. Dr G M Craig argues that it may be inappropriate and misjudged.[l]

Enshrined in UK law and practice (subject to a number of exceptions) is the principle of sanctity of life and the duty, where possible and appropriate, to preserve life. However, the courts have come to recognise that some quality of life is so poor and hopeless that it does not warrant further attempts to maintain it and therefore that it is lawful to allow the patient to die. Sometimes the patient may take this decision and if he is lucid and capable then his refusal to consent to treatment which his doctors consider appropriate and for his benefit may be valid and lawful and should be respected.

THE LAW COMMISSION'S PROPOSED GUIDELINES

Guidance is to be found in the Law Commission's Consultation Paper 129, Part II paras 12 and 13 in its proposals as to best interest criteria. Consideration should be given to:

12 (1)   the ascertainable past and present wishes and feelings (considered in the light of his or her understanding at the time) of the incapacitated person;
   (2)   whether there is an alternative to the proposed treatment, and in particular whether there is an alternative which is more conservative or which is less intrusive or restrictive;
   (3)   the factors which the incapacitated person might be expected to consider if able to do so, including the likely effect of the treatment on the person's life expectancy, health, happiness, freedom and dignity.
13   The interests of people other than the incapacitated person should not be considered except to the extent that they have a bearing on the incapacitated person's individual interests.[m]

In *Airedale NHS Trust* v *Bland* the withdrawal of medical treatment (in this case artificial hydration and nutrition) was held to take the form of a legal omission rather than commission and was lawful *in that case.*

Each of the successive courts who heard the arguments in *Airedale NHS Trust* v *Bland* emphasised that the issues under discussion and review bore no relation to euthanasia. In particular, *R* v *Cox* was distinguished and many of the judges involved were anxious for Parliament to review the position. However, the Parliamentary Committee of the House of Lords did not suggest any changes in the law (see above). The lobby in favour of legalising euthanasia with safeguards is likely to continue its efforts to achieve a change in the law.

REFERENCES

a   For a history of the development of Dutch medical practice of euthanasia and the legal position, see:
   Sluyters B 1989 Euthanasia in the Netherlands (The Baron de Lancey Lecture 1988, Council of Legal Education) Medico-Legal Journal 1989:1:34

Brahams D 1990 Euthanasia in the Netherlands. The Lancet i:591.
See also Sheldon T 1994 Dutch watch euthanasia on television, and Dillner L
1994 Relatives keener on euthanasia than patients, both in British Medical
Journal 309: 1107

b   Devlin P 1985 Easing the passing. Bodley Head, London: 165
c   Ibid: 171 et seq., quoting direction to the jury
d   Ibid
e   Select Committee on Medical Ethics 1994 (HL Paper 21) Vol.I: Report; Vol.II:
    Oral evidence; Vol.III: Written evidence. HMSO, London
f   Ibid
g   A review is likely (and overdue) on the issue of whether a conviction of murder
    should continue automatically to carry a mandatory life sentence without
    opportunity for judicial discretion
h   Brahams D 1992 Criminality and compassion. Law Society's Gazette 35:2
i   The charge against Dr Arthur was reduced to attempted murder during the trial
    in response to the Prosecution's evidential difficulties. See Brahams D, Brahams
    M 1981 R v Arthur — a suitable case for treatment? Law Society's Gazette 25
    November 1981
j   Ibid. See also Brahams D 1981. The Lancet ii:1981
k   Ognall J A right to die? Some medico-legal reflections. Medical Law Reports
    62:165
l   Craig G M 1994 On withholding nutrition and hydration in the terminally ill:
    has the palliative medicine gone too far? Journal of Medical Ethics 20:139–143
m   For discussion see Brahams D 1992 Criminality and compassion. Law Society's
    Gazette 35:2. For similar discussion of Airedale NHS Trust v Bland while at
    Court of Appeal level, see Brahams D 1992 Of life and death. Law Society's
    Gazette 46:3. For a discussion of the legal and ethical issues see also Mason J K,
    McCall Smith A 1991 Law and medical ethics, 4th edn. Butterworths, London;
    Brazier M 1992 Medicine, patients and the law, 2nd edn. Penguin, London

10. Organ donation

Robert Parker

INTRODUCTION

From the eleventh century, when the patron saints of transplantation, Cosmos and Damien, performed the first transplant, until the beginning of this century, the field of transplantation and organ donation was looked upon as having science fiction overtones. Cosmos and Damien transplanted the leg of a slave who had recently died, to replace a cancerous leg, but unfortunately the outcome of the operation was not recorded. In the 19th century, a Russian soldier was excommunicated after he received the first bone transplant taken from the skull of a dog, and this is probably the first 'civil action' that took place over a transplant. It was not until this century that transplantation became a recognised therapeutic intervention with the first corneal transplant in 1905, the kidney in 1954, heart valves in 1962, liver in 1963 and heart in 1967.

According to data published in 1994 by the Kings Fund Institute[a] there were over 20 000 kidney transplants, 6000 liver transplants and 4200 heart transplants performed in 1993 in the world's leading cadaveric transplant countries. The figures would have been considerably higher if data from Russia and China had been included. In the first 9 months of 1994, United Kingdom Transplant Support Services Agency reported 699 cadaveric solid organ donors (a 1% increase over the previous year) which had enabled 1303 kidney transplants, 236 heart transplants, 40 heart and lung transplants, 88 lung transplants and 477 liver transplants to be performed.[b] Overall the number of transplants increased by 3% compared with the previous year. However, in the UK there were still nearly 5000 people on the waiting list for a kidney transplant and several hundred each for heart, heart and lung, and liver transplants. At the present time organ donation is controlled by three Acts:

- Human Tissue Act 1961
- Corneal Tissue Act 1986
- Human Organ Transplants Act 1989

99

Before considering these acts it is necessary to look at what is death for the purposes of organ donation and the donating process.

DEFINITION OF DEATH

There is no statutory definition of death in English law, so for transplants it is usually accepted as brain stem death. In 1980 a Revision Committee on Criminal Law decided that it would only give the current view for that year and that this would need regular updating, thereby making it impractical to legislate. Both Skegg[c] and Jennett[d] have put forward the case that death should be defined, to prevent the transplant surgeon facing a charge of murder, as has happened in Japan. There, the concept of brain stem death is not accepted, unless accompanied by cardiac or respiratory death. The diagnosis of brain death is clearly defined in the Report of the Working Party on behalf of the Health Departments of Great Britain and Northern Ireland on Cadaveric Organs for Transplantation.[e] This report lists a series of tests that must be performed to establish brain death and must be repeated after a suitable time by a second medical practitioner. Both practitioners must have been qualified for at least five years and be independent of the transplant team. A group of patients where it is difficult to ascertain brain stem death are anacephalic infants where there is little higher brain activity. The Medical Royal College Working Party on Organ Transplantation from Neonates in 1988[f] suggested that no organs should be removed during the first 7 days of life because of the difficulty of defining death in these individuals, and the view was expressed that death occurred when spontaneous breathing had stopped, and this had been certified by two independent medical practitioners.

DEFINITION OF ORGANS AND TISSUES

The 1989 Human Organ Transplants Act defines 'organ' as any part of a human body consisting of a structured arrangement of tissues which, if wholly removed, cannot be replicated by the body.[g] From this it is clear that kidneys, liver, heart, lungs and pancreas are definitely organs, but the status of bone, cornea and tendon are less clear in this respect and have been omitted from the Human Organ Transplant Regulations forms, although heart valves are included on the forms. For the purpose of the 1989 Act, skin is excluded as an organ due to its ability to replicate.

Donation of organs and tissues

Great Britain has an opting-in system for organ donation in common with the majority of the world's countries. The basis of this system is the Donor Card, which, according to the Department of Health's data, 30% of the population possess. Up to 35% of these people, however, do not carry it with them. 70% of people have stated that they were willing to donate their organs after their death.[h] The Government has introduced the National Transplant Register to try to improve the total number of potential donors by having all the data on computer and including the request on driving licence applications. Some countries including Belgium, France and Israel have an opting-out system where there is a central computer file based on National Insurance or National Identity numbers of people who do not want their organs used after their death. Several attempts have been made to introduce this system in Britain, including a Private Members Bill in 1984, but to date all have been unsuccessful.

There is no minimum age for having a donor card in Britain. With the safeguard as laid down in the Human Tissue Act 1961 of having to ask a surviving relative (who would in these cases have to be the parent or guardian), there would appear to be no reason why a child who was competent should not be able to carry a donor card and have his wishes respected. 50% of organ donors are in intensive care units and have died from intracranial pathology. To try to increase donor numbers, various hospitals led by Royal Devon & Exeter Hospital started elective ventilation of certain patients in 1988. The purpose of this was to maintain patients with poor prognosis in a viable state for donation of organs. The ethics of this led to considerable discussion over a 5-year period until Mr Tom Sackville, the Minister for Health, ruled in 1994 that this procedure was not acceptable.[i]

Human Tissue Act 1961

This Act permits the person in legal possession of the body to allow parts of the body of a deceased person to be removed for transplantation providing he has no reason to believe that the deceased had objected to it or that surviving relatives object to it.[j] There is no agreed ownership of a cadaver under English Law. If the person dies under conditions where their death is notified to the coroner, the latter has jurisdiction over the body and is therefore assumed to be in legal possession of it. The Human Tissue Act requires that if there is reason to believe that an inquest or a coroner's post mortem *may* be required, the consent of the coroner *must* be obtained prior to the removal of any tissues. If the person dies in hospital or nursing home the Act entrusts the legal possession of the body to the Administrator of the institution until it is claimed by the next of kin. Funeral directors, though in physical possession of the body, are not deemed to have legal possession of the cadaver. The Act also states that the person in legal possession must make such reasonable enquiry as may be practical to ascertain lack of objection from any surviving relative. Most transplant co-ordinators will only ask the next of kin this question and will not make efforts to contact other relatives as the term 'any relative' is extremely vague. As there is a time limit for the removal of organs, consideration is required of what is meant by the words 'may be practical', and in a number of cases organs have been removed as no relatives have been found within an agreed period defined normally by the coroner. It is practice, but not legally tested, that the wishes of the parents and spouse from whom the donor had been separated take precedence over the wishes of the person with whom the donor had cohabited for a number of years. The Act does not state that the lack of objection of the relatives must be stated in writing, therefore verbal permission is often used with the requester making a note of this in an appropriate document, (e.g. the patient's notes if the donor died in hospital). The Act does allow, without consulting the relatives, removal of parts of the body if the donor during his last illness had expressed this wish in the presence of two witnesses. Donor cards do not need witnesses and, as many donors die suddenly from brain causes rendering them unconscious, they are unable to express their wish to donate in front of two witnesses during their final illness.

Corneal Tissue Act 1986

The main purpose of this Act is to allow suitably qualified persons, who are not medical practitioners, to remove eyes or parts of eyes, primarily for corneal transplantation.[k] The persons must be employees of a health authority and be trained by a medical practitioner. They must be satisfied that life is extinct, and corneal donors have usually undergone cardiac and respiratory death, as well as brain stem death, at the time of removal, which is normally between 2 and 18 hours after death.

Human Organ Transplants Act 1989

This Act together with its accompanying regulations was designed to prohibit dealing in human organs, to control transplants between unrelated living donors and to provide information about transplant operations.[g] The Act was prompted by advertisements inserted by doctors from Britain in a Turkish newspaper offering to pay for kidneys for transplantation.[1] A small number of people 'agreed' to have one of their kidneys removed and these were subsequently transplanted into private foreign patients in a London clinic. The Act prohibits the sale of human tissue and provides criminal sanctions for the donor, advertiser, or surgeon removing or implanting such organs. The practice of selling organs from executed criminals, which occurs in China, is thus illegal and attempted importation of such organs into Britain would be unlawful. The Act allows hospitals to charge for the costs of removing, transporting and preserving organs and the repayment of expenses and loss of earnings of live donors. With whole organs it is generally theatre operating time and transport that is charged, while with tissue (e.g. bone and heart valves) hospitals tend to fix a processing charge. The Belgian government has determined a processing charge nationwide and such a system may be implemented in this country because of the differences in processing charges levied by hospitals.

The second part of the Act prohibits a transplant of an organ from a living individual to another if they are not genetically related unless the operation is approved by the Unrelated Live Transplant Regulatory Authority. The commonest organ transplant being referred to the Authority is the heart, where the heart from a heart and lung transplant recipient is needed for transplant into a patient requiring heart replacement and the aortic and pulmonary heart valves from the second recipient are then transplanted into two other individuals. In these cases the Authority must be satisfied that there is no inducement offered to the donor and that the request has been made by the medical practitioner with clinical responsibility for the donor. In other cases where the organ removal is not part of the treatment of the donor, such as a kidney transplant from a fit unrelated individual, the latter must also be counselled by a medical practitioner, have the risks outlined and his rights explained.

The final section of the Act and Regulations sets up a database of organ donation and transplant, whereby the doctor who removes any organ must complete a form giving details of himself, the donor (live or cadaveric), the organs removed, the time and place of removal and their destination. Similarly the transplanting surgeon must complete a second form giving details of himself, the recipient and his status, the organs transplanted and time and place of transplantation. Copies of both forms must be sent to the United Kingdom Transplant Support Service Authority, working as agents for the Department of Health.

Ownership of tissue

In the Nuffield Council on Bioethics Report, 'Human tissue: ethical and legal issues', the subject of tissue ownership is raised. It is stated that English law is silent on whether parts of a body are property but that the traditional view is that they are not, so that the donor has no right to them providing appropriate consent had been obtained. For the same reason the user of the tissue and the recipient of the tissue have possessory rights but this does not mean they can do whatever they like with the tissue. It would probably be illegal to use tissue for research if the only permission that had been sought was for transplantation.

Liability

The Human Organ Transplants Act 1989 is the only one of the three Acts concerning donation and transplantation that states the penalties for not complying with the Act. It also states that the organisation (and therefore its chief executive) can be guilty of the offence as well as any individual. The Human Tissue Act 1961 and the Corneal Tissue Act 1986 are far less clear in what criminal offence is committed if the provisions are not followed. The Kings Fund Report's authors state[a] that the only offence would be the general common law disobedience to a statute, but that this had been criticised by the Law Commission in 1976[m] and Horseferry Road Justices in 1987.[n] If the donor requires a Coroner's post mortem or an inquest, there is the possibility of being considered to have obstructed the Coroner at common law if the Coroner's consent was not obtained prior to the removal of tissue.

Where tissue is being processed, in the case of heart valves, bone and skin, the organisation undertaking this must conform to relevant standards according to the Consumer Protection Act 1987.[o] At the present time there are no written UK national standards, but the British Association of Tissue Banks and their European counterparts are currently drafting these. The Food and Drug Administration in America have approved a standard for the USA.[p]

Most of the tissue for transplantation would be covered by the development risk case (see Ch. 14) and the processor would only be liable if negligence could be proved, for example if he had not observed all the precautions and testing in force at the time of preparation.

The future

When the success of the UK National Transplant Register is assessed in a few years' time, it will then be appropriate to discuss whether Britain should adopt an opting-out procedure for transplantation. It is also possible that the European Union may try to rationalise donation procedures, to integrate the legal aspects of organ transplantation throughout the Union. An alternative to this would be 'required-request' legislation which would compel a hospital to ask the relative about organ donation. This could possibly be extended in the case of tissue donation to include coroner's officers or pathologists for cases brought in dead. One problem with this method is that the approach to the relatives could be forced and make donation less likely.

Genetic engineering is now allowing the breeding of transgenic pigs from which organs could be transplanted with low risk of rejection, but the subject raises a number of ethical issues, most of which would not be covered by present legislation. It would also seem likely that there will be transplantable artificial hearts within the next decade, but prosthetic kidneys, livers and lungs small and reliable enough to implant are still a considerable way off.

REFERENCES

a   New B, Solomon M, Dingwall R, McHale J 1994 A question of give and take. Improving the supply of donor organs for transplantation. Kings Fund Institute Research Report 18. Kings Fund Institute, London

b   United Kingdom Transplant Support Service Authority 1994 Transplant update. UKTSSA, Bristol

c   Skegg P D G 1976 The case for a statutory 'definition of death'. Journal of Medical Ethics 2: 190–192

d   Jennett B 1977 Diagnosis of brain death. Journal of Medical Ethics 3:4–5

e   Working Party on behalf of the Health Department of Great Britain and Northern Ireland 1983 Transplantation: a code of practice including the diagnosis of brain death. Department of Health and Social Security, London

f   Working Party on Organ Transplantation from Neonates 1988 Report. Conference of Medical Royal Colleges and their Faculties in the UK, London

g   Human Organ Transplants Act 1989. HMSO, London
h   Department of Health 1992 Research surveys of Great Britain: omnibus survey.
    Department of Health, London
i   NHS Executive Circular 1994 HSG(94)41
j   Human Tissue Act 1961. HMSO, London
k   Corneal Tissue Act 1986. HMSO, London
l   World Health Organization Circular 1988 WH40.13
m   Law Commission 1976 Report on Conspiracy and Criminal Law Reform. HC
    Papers 1975/6 No. 176: 140. Law Commission, London
n   *R* v *Horseferry Road Justices ex p IBA* [1987]; Mason J K 1992 Organ donation
    and transplantation. In: Dyer C (ed) Doctors, patients and the law. Blackwell,
    London
o   Consumer Protection Act 1987. HMSO, London
p   US Government Code of Federal Regulations 21, part 812

FURTHER READING

Nuffield Council on Bioethics 1995 Human tissue: ethical and legal issues. Nuffield
    Council on Bioethics, London

11. Abortion and reproductive health

Catherine James

INTRODUCTION

Few issues in medicine generate such heated discussion as abortion; technological advances have opened up possibilities for the creation of human life in circumstances unimagined even a decade ago; and women's own attitudes to pregnancy and contraception have changed profoundly.

ABORTION

Common law references to the offence of abortion can be traced back to the 12th century but the present law is found in Section 58 and Section 59 of the Offences against the Person Act 1861 and the Abortion Act 1967 (as amended). It is a criminal offence for any person: '. . . with intent to procure the miscarriage of any woman, whether she be or be not with child . . .' unless this is carried out within the conditions laid down by the Abortion Act.

There is much legal debate over the definition of 'miscarriage'. Some authorities[a] hold the view that as soon as the ovum is fertilised it is 'carried' in the woman's body. This would effectively make post-coital contraception illegal unless undertaken in accordance with the Abortion Act (as amended). Others[b,c] favour implantation as the starting point since it is only then that the fetus is truly 'carried' in the uterus and thus capable of 'miscarriage'. In practice, following the Attorney General's statement[d] in 1983, which favoured the 'implantation' argument, no prosecution will result against medical practitioners who provide post-coital contraception aimed at its prevention. A note of caution is appropriate here. The Attorney General's ruling was given with specific reference to the 'morning after' pill and has been interpreted as applying also to the post-coital insertion of an intrauterine contraceptive device (IUD), prior to implantation of the fertilized ovum, another method available at that time. It is not necessarily the case that other forms of post-coital contraception more recently introduced (e.g. the anti-progestogen, mifepristone) will be regarded in the same light if it seems their effect is mediated by abortifacient properties rather than interceptive intervention. The use of mifepristone for the medical induction of abortion is permitted through approved clinics under section 37(3) of the Human Fertilisation and Embryology Act 1990.

The legalisation of abortion in certain defined circumstances was introduced in England and Wales within the framework of the Abortion Act 1967. Prior to that, the Offences Against the Person Act 1861 (referred to above) had been enforced rigorously although in the famous case of *R* v *Bourne* [1938][1] a gynaecologist was acquitted of a charge of criminal abortion on the grounds that he had acted to preserve the life of the mother. The definition of 'life' in this instance was a broad one, ensuring that the mother did not become 'a physical and mental wreck'.

Originally, the Abortion Act 1967 permitted a pregnancy to be terminated provided *two* (in an emergency, one) registered medical practitioners were of the opinion, formed in good faith, that either (1) the continuance of the pregnancy would involve greater risk to the life of the mother or of injury to her or her existing children's physical or mental health or (2) that there was a substantial risk of fetal handicap. Whilst that general framework remains, amendments to the Abortion Act made by the Human Fertilisation and Embryology Act 1990 have introduced significant changes. In order to understand these changes a brief historical resumé is required. The common law of homicide can apply only once a baby has been expelled from its mother's body, and so in order to protect the life of a child in utero who was considered to be 'capable of being born alive' the Infant Life (Preservation) Act 1929 introduced the offence of 'child destruction'. The Abortion Act 1967 did not alter the provisions of the Infant Life (Preservation) Act — it merely created a defence to prosecution provided a pregnancy was terminated in accordance with the Act's provisions.

For many years 28 weeks was taken as the presumed gestation at which a fetus would be 'capable of being born alive' even after neonatal advances rendered an earlier gestation more logical. The amendments to the Abortion Act that came into effect in April

---

1 *R* v *Bourne* [1938] 3 All ER: 615–621

1991 now reflect contemporary standards such that termination in the majority of cases is subject to *an upper limit of 24 weeks* (see Box 11.1). However, amendments have extended the period in which termination may be performed in some cases. Where continuation of the pregnancy may result in grave permanent harm/death of the mother or where there is substantial risk of severe fetal handicap, termination can be undertaken *irrespective of gestation*. Such a pregnancy may thus be terminated legally up to term, made possible now by the specific exclusion of these cases from the remit of the Infant Life (Preservation) Act 1929. But this protects the obstetrician only as far as an *unborn* child is concerned. If 'termination' results in a live birth with subsequent death or handicap, criminal charges for murder or manslaughter might be considered.

Box 11.1 Grounds for medical termination of pregnancy

Abortion Act 1967 (as amended by Section 37 of the Human Fertilisation and Embryology Act 1990):

a. that the pregnancy has not exceeded its twenty-fourth week and that the continuance of the pregnancy would involve risk, greater than if the pregnancy were terminated, of injury to the physical or mental health of the pregnant woman or any existing children of her family; **or**
b. that the termination is necessary to prevent grave permanent injury to the physical or mental health of the pregnant woman; **or**
c. that the continuance of the pregnancy would involve risk to the life of the pregnant woman, greater than if the pregnancy were terminated; **or**
d. that there is a substantial risk that if the child were born it would suffer from such physical or mental abnormalities as to be seriously handicapped.

Selective reduction of multiple pregnancy has been given recognition within the amended legislation provided it is undertaken for one of the grounds for which termination of the pregnancy as a whole would be lawful (see above).

Some health professionals have religious or ethical objections to abortion and the Abortion Act 1967 does contain a clause that allows non-participation on grounds of conscience. How far does that 'non-participation' extend? In 1987 Mrs Janaway, a secretary with a local health authority, sought judicial review to overturn her employer's decision to terminate her employment because she had refused to type a letter of referral for an abortion on grounds of conscience. Her application was refused and in 1988 the House of Lords dismissed her appeal.[2] It was held that 'participation' meant 'taking part in treatment' and not merely arrangements preliminary to such treatment.

On occasion there may be a difference of opinion between the prospective parents as to whether a pregnancy should be terminated. The cases of *Paton* v *Trustees of BPAS and another* [1978][3] and *C and another* v *S and another* [1987][4] established that a father had no authority in law to prevent the mother undergoing such a procedure nor could the fetus in utero be a party to an action whilst it was unborn.

Modern methods of abortion may not necessarily require the intervention of a medical practitioner throughout. When termination is medically induced it may be a nurse who continues the treatment initiated by a doctor. However the Abortion Act 1967 protects against prosecution only 'when a pregnancy is terminated by a registered medical practitioner'. Although the then Department of Health and Social Security (DHSS) issued guidance to nurses indicating that their involvement in such terminations was legal, the Royal College of Nursing challenged this interpretation. In 1980 the House of Lords ruled that, provided a doctor prescribed the treatment for termination, remained in charge throughout, and the treatment was carried out according to his directions, *any person* taking part in the termination was entitled to the protection offered by the Abortion Act against prosecution.[5]

Finally, practitioners should remember that they have a statutory obligation to notify any termination that they have undertaken to the Department of Health within seven days and the appropriate certificate must be retained in the medical records for 3 years. Any person who 'wilfully contravenes' or 'wilfully fails to comply' with these requirements under Section 2 of the Abortion Act 1967 may find themselves liable on summary conviction to a fine of up to £5000.

2 *Janaway* v *Salford Health Authority* [1988] 3 All ER: 1079–1084
3 *Paton* v *Trustees of BPAS and another* [1978] 2 All ER: 987–992
4 *C and another* v *S and another* [1987] 1 All ER: 1230–44
5 *Royal College of Nursing of the United Kingdom* v *Department of Health and Social Security* [1981] 1 All ER: 545–578

CONTRACEPTION

Contraception has never been banned in the UK as it has in some countries but particular medicolegal difficulties arise in two areas.

The young person

In the words of Lord Templeman in the case of *Gillick*, '. . . There are many things a girl under 16 needs to practise but sex is not one of them'.[6] Clearly the teenagers of Britain are not following Lord Templeman's advice since one in five girls has had sexual intercourse before the age of 16 and one in 100 becomes pregnant.[e] Fear that doctors will not respect their confidences deters many young women from seeking contraceptive advice. The Family Law Reform Act 1969 reduced the age of presumed consent for medical treatment to 16 years but does this mean that doctors have the freedom to see and treat those *under 16* without parental involvement as discretion and the maturity of the young person dictates?

This was the issue that lay at the heart of the Gillick case, which had its origins in a DHSS circular published in 1974 and revised in 1980. This advised that if a girl under 16 did not wish her parents to be told of her request for contraception then those wishes should be respected, though every effort should be made to encourage parental involvement in her decision. Mrs Gillick, the mother of four daughters under 16, sought an assurance from her local health authority that her daughters would not be given contraceptive or abortion advice without her prior knowledge and agreement. This assurance was not forthcoming and so Mrs Gillick sought a court declaration that the DHSS advice was unlawful and wrong. Her case eventually reached the House of Lords who by a margin of three to two upheld the DHSS advice. The judgment, given in 1985, can be summarised thus: a doctor would be justified in providing contraceptive advice to a girl under 16 provided he was satisfied that she could understand his advice; he could not persuade her to involve her parents; she was likely to have sexual intercourse and that, unless contraceptive advice was given, her physical and/or mental health was likely to suffer.

The way was thus cleared for doctors to provide contraceptive advice to young girls under the age of 16 without parental consent.

---

6 *Gillick* v *West Norfolk and Wisbech Area Health Authority and Another* [1985] 3 All ER: 402–437

Further legislation, particularly the Children Act 1989 with its concept of parental responsibility rather than parental right, has further reinforced that concept.

It is a crime under the Sexual Offences Act 1956 for a man to have sexual intercourse with a girl under 16 irrespective of consent. The Act further states that a prosecution could be brought against any person who causes or encourages the 'commission of unlawful sexual intercourse with a girl for whom (the) accused is responsible'. Does this make a doctor vulnerable if he offers contraceptive advice? In the Gillick judgment the Law Lords held by a majority that no offence had been committed. This view was not unanimous and the doctor who cannot show that his decision was based on a careful assessment may still be vulnerable under criminal law and before the General Medical Council (see Chapter 2).

The mentally handicapped patient

Control of fertility in the mentally handicapped is a problem that is often brought to the medical practitioner. The legal position regarding permanent contraception has been clarified by the House of Lords decision in the case of *F* v *West Berkshire Health Authority*[7] It was held that an adult woman incapable of giving informed consent by virtue of mental impairment could be sterilised, provided the operation was considered to be in her best interests. This is defined as treatment carried out to 'either save the patient's life or ensure improvement or prevent deterioration in the patient's physical or mental health'. What constitutes best interests is a matter to be decided by the doctor in accordance with good professional practice as defined by a reasonable body of medical opinion. In practice an application should be made to the Court for a declaration that the proposed procedure is lawful in an individual case. The steps to be followed are set out in the Department of Health's Circular HC(90)22 revised in 1992.[f] Where sterilisation is not the primary purpose of surgery, as in the case of a hysterectomy for intractable menorrhagia, Court approval need not be obtained,[8] provided other less radical treatments are not appropriate and the recommendation is supported by two consultant colleagues. Termination of pregnancy also requires no prelimi-

7 *F* v *West Berkshire Health Authority and Another* (Mental Health Commission intervening) [1989] 2 All ER: 545–571
8 *Re E (a minor) (medical treatment)* [1991] 7 BMLR: 117–119. Butterworths, London

nary Court approval provided it is performed in accordance with the Abortion Act and in the best interests of the patient.[9] No powers exist under the Mental Health Act 1983 to sanction such a procedure when the patient herself is incapable of giving informed consent[10] and neither can a relative consent on the patient's behalf.

Of course the clinician's opinion should be documented carefully in the patient's medical records and where there is any doubt in an individual case medicolegal advice should be sought.

INFERTILITY

Infertility affects approximately one in 10 couples. In vitro fertilisation (IVF), embryo storage and transplantation, egg donation and womb leasing have offered hope to childless couples in circumstances that would until recently have seemed impossible. When much is offered to those in desperate need their interests require protection from exploitation. Such protection was initially provided by the Voluntary Licensing Authority, later the Interim Licensing Authority, set up in 1985 to monitor and license all embryo research and IVF treatment. This body was replaced in 1991 by the Human Fertilisation and Embryology Authority (HFEA), a statutory group set up to regulate the legislation regarding infertility treatment introduced by the Human Fertilisation and Embryology Act 1990. As of August 1991 IVF, artificial insemination by a donor (AID), donor gamete intrafallopian transfer (GIFT), egg donation and intravaginal culture (IVC) can only be performed in centres licensed by the HFEA. Initially the very restrictive confidentiality provisions of the Act prevented a licensed practitioner from disclosing information about his patient that related to the fertility services given. Effectively this barred the direct exchange of information with the patient's own general practitioner and other non-licensed clinicians. It also deprived the licensed practitioner of the right to defend himself should litigation or complaints arise. These problems have now largely been resolved following the introduction of the Human Fertilisation and Embryology (Disclosure of Information) Act in July 1992 but consent for assisted conception has specific requirements set down in the 1990 Act (as now amended). The HFEA offers guidance in its Code of Practice[g] on the workings of the Act and its practical interpretation.

---

9 *Re G* The Times: 31 January 1991
10 *T v T and Another* [1988] 1 All ER: 613–625

Scientific advance in the field of assisted conception has brought with it a number of ethical, social and medicolegal dilemmas. Embryo research is one such area of controversy that has become the subject of legislation. This may be conducted only under licence from the HFEA and only up to 14 days post-fertilisation.

The HFEA consults widely when contentious issues arise. In 1993 it canvassed views on whether sex selection should be permitted as part of an infertility clinic's licensed activities. It then approved in principle the use of sex selection techniques for medical reasons in cases where a woman risks having a child with a life threatening sex-linked disease. In 1994 the Authority sought opinion on the use of donated ovarian tissue, including that from aborted fetuses, in the treatment of infertility. It concluded that for *treatment* purposes it would be acceptable to use tissue *only* from live donors. However, for *embryo research* the Authority supported the use of tissue both from live donors and cadavers or fetuses.

What then of the couple who cannot achieve a pregnancy even with in vitro techniques? Is the option of surrogacy open to them? Surrogacy without payment is not a criminal offence but the Surrogacy Arrangements Act 1985 prevents the setting up of surrogacy on a commercial basis. Its restrictions are limited to agencies or individuals whose purpose is to make a profit out of such activities. No offence in relation to surrogacy is committed if the surrogate mother herself accepts payment or if the commissioning couple offer payment to her, although all three may be guilty of an offence under the Adoption Act 1976.[h]

CONCLUSION

There are unlikely to be any major changes to the law on abortion and assisted conception in the near future, given the wide-ranging nature of the Human Fertilisation and Embryology Act 1990. Some minor amendments are introduced on a regular basis to deal with such matters as legal parenthood when genetic and natural parents may differ but these do not touch on the fundamental moral issues of the right to life; whose rights should take precedence and who should exercise those rights. Whilst debate is certain to continue, the present law in Britain is unambiguous in the following respect: its view that the fetus has no rights until it is born, that the severely handicapped fetus has no protection against destruction at any gestation, and that ultimately the choice for termination rests not with the fetus, be it normal or abnormal, nor with its parents, but with the medical profession.

ACKNOWLEDGMENT

I am most grateful to Mr Ian Barker of Messrs. Hempsons for his advice and assistance in the preparation of this article.

REFERENCES

a   Keown J 1984 Miscarriage: a medico legal analysis. Criminal Law Review 1984: 604–614
b   Williams G 1983 Textbook on criminal law, 2nd edn: 294–295. Stevens, London
c   Mason J K 1988 Human life and medical practice: 90–92. Edinburgh University Press, Edinburgh
d   House of Commons: Written answers, 10 May 1983: cols 236–237. Hansard, London
e   Department of Health 1993 Health and personal social statistics for England: 13. HMSO, London
f   Department of Health 1992 Circular HC(90)22 / HSG(92)32, Patient consent to examination and treatment. Department of Health, London
g   Human Fertilisation and Embryology Authority 1993 Code of practice. Human Fertilisation and Embryology Authority, London
h   Brazier M 1992 Assisted conception. In: Brazier M 1992 Medicine, patients and the law, 2nd edn: 283. Penguin, London

FURTHER READING

Brazier M 1992 Medicine, patients and the law, 2nd edn. Penguin, London
Dyer C (ed) 1992 Doctors, patients and the law. Blackwell Scientific, London
Morgan D, Lee R G 1991 Blackstone's guide to the Human Fertilisation and Embryology Act 1990. Blackstone Press, London
Templeton A A, Cusine D (eds) 1990 Reproductive medicine and the law. Churchill Livingstone, Edinburgh

12. The Children Act 1989

Allan Levy QC

INTRODUCTION

The Children Act 1989 is landmark legislation by any standards. Even allowing for political hyperbole, there is some force in the observation of one minister, when introducing the bill in Parliament, that it is the most comprehensive and far-reaching reform of child law in living memory. The Act has 108 sections and 15 schedules, and over 30 sets of Rules and Regulations. The long title of the statute gives an indication of its comprehensive nature: 'An Act to reform the law relating to children; to provide for local authority services for children in need and others; to amend the law with respect to children's homes, community homes, voluntary homes and voluntary organisations; to make provision with respect to fostering, child minding and day care for young children, and adoption; and for connected purposes'. The legislation was passed in 1989 but not implemented until October 1991.[a]

Background

In the early 1980s it became abundantly clear that reform of the law regarding children was a priority. Parts of it were ultimately and accurately described in Parliament as 'confusing, piecemeal, outdated, often unfair and in important respects ineffective . . . most notably when it comes to our ability to protect children at risk'. In 1982 the House of Commons Social Services Select Committee began consideration of the issue, and concluded in 1984 that a review of child care law was overdue. In January 1987 following a Consultation Paper and a Review, the Government published a White Paper, 'The Law on Child Care and Family Services'.[b] The key points in the proposals included an improvement of the powers to protect children from abuse and neglect, and a more thorough and fair testing of orders to transfer to the local authority parental rights, to make sure this really was in the best interests of the child.

Later in 1987 the Cleveland affair, which led to a public inquiry and the influential Cleveland Report,[c] burst on an unsuspecting Britain. This alerted the public to the problems of diagnosing child sexual abuse and the real dangers of overreaction to suspected abuse. A large number of children, over a relatively short space of time, were removed from their parents in Cleveland, following allegations that the children had been sexually abused. The allegations were to a significant extent based upon a controversial medical test relating to physical signs of sexual abuse: reflex anal dilatation. There were considerable delays in the cases coming to court and there was great concern about the medical, social work and legal procedures and practices adopted. The comprehensive Report produced after a judicial inquiry acted as a substantial trigger to reform of the law.

A succession of inquiries[d] into the deaths of children resulting from child abuse further fuelled the impetus to reform. Critical comments from the European Court of Human Rights in Strasbourg in a number of cases concerning child care issues[1] also helped. In addition the decision of the House of Lords in the case of *Gillick*[2] was a considerable influence. Central to the case was the question whether a girl under 16 had the legal capacity to consent to a medical examination and treatment. The law lords held that she had the capacity, including the capacity to consent to contraceptive treatment, if she had sufficient maturity and intelligence to understand the nature and implications of the proposed treatment. This decision, essentially about children's rights regarding decision-making, had a major effect on the debate about law reform.

Parallel with the review of child care law, the Law Commission had carried out its own review of child law in respect of the 'private' law of custody, access, guardianship and wardship. It produced a number of working papers and a final Report.[e] The draft Bill which the Law Commission annexed to its Report covered the reviews of both child care law and 'private' child law. This helpfully led to all the public and private law being gathered together in one place, the Children Act 1989, enabling common principles and remedies to be formulated, where possible, regarding both private and public law.

---

1 *R* v *O, R and W* [1988] 2 FLR 445
2 *Gillick* v *West Norfolk and Wisbech AHA* [1986] AC 112

MAIN POLICIES OF THE ACT

Welfare

Section 1(1) of the Act provides that when a court determines any question with respect to the upbringing of a child, the child's welfare shall be the paramount consideration. The limiting words are important and it is not correct to say that the Children Act 1989 always puts the welfare of the child as the paramount consideration. Certain provisions within the Act apply different tests. A court being asked by a local authority, for example, to consider making a care or supervision order under section 31 (see below) must first decide if the precise threshold condition as to significant harm is proved and the welfare principle plays no part in the exercise. If the condition is proved then the welfare principle comes into play, and section 1(3) provides a check-list of matters to be taken into account. These include the ascertainable wishes and feelings of the child concerned (considered in the light of his age and understanding), his physical, emotional and educational needs, and the range of powers available to the court under the Act in the proceedings in question.

Family care

It is fundamental to the legislation that whenever possible children should be brought up and cared for in their own families. The Act's philosophy is that the child in need can be helped most effectively if the local authority, working in partnership with the parents, provides a range and level of services appropriate to the child's needs. Complementary to this approach is the belief that the state, in the form of the local authority, should not be permitted to control a child's life in any way unless strict statutory criteria are met and a court order obtained. Any possible administrative route into care, for instance a parental rights resolution, has been abolished.

Parental responsibility

The Act introduced the concept of parental responsibility. This is defined in section 3(1) as 'any of the rights, duties, powers, responsibilities and authority which by law a parent of a child has in relation to the child and his property'. Although the definition refers to rights, the intention of the legislation is to emphasise the child as a person and not a possession. Powers and duties given to parents exist in order that they can carry out their responsibilities.

No order

The Law Commission considered that orders were sometimes unnecessary and might discourage parties from negotiating arrangements or agreements. In addition an order might deter a parent from remaining involved with a child after separation or divorce. Accordingly, section 1(5) states that the court must not make an order unless it considers that to do so would be better for the child than making no order at all.

Delay

The court must have regard to the general principle that delay in determining a question with respect to the upbringing of a child is likely to prejudice the child's welfare.[f] This attempts to meet one of the main criticisms of proceedings relating to children. Rules of court deal with the particular timetables to be followed.

Contact

When children are removed from home under a court order by a local authority, contact with the parents should be maintained, except where it would be dangerous or harmful to the child. Section 34 of the Act deals in detail with parental contact with children in care.

Services for children in need

A local authority has statutory duties to provide services for children in need. Schedule 2 of the Act sets out an extensive list of services for families and in respect of children looked after by local authorities. Headings in the schedule include 'Prevention of neglect and abuse', 'Provision of accommodation in order to protect child' and 'Provision for children living with their families'.

Court structure

The Act provides an integrated and improved court structure, with all the courts in essence having the same remedies and powers. This principle was important if the previously unsatisfactory practice of forum-shopping (i.e. having in certain circumstances a number of different jurisdictions to choose from and litigate in) was to be ended.

Aims of the Act

The aims of the Act, therefore, are to simplify, to reform, to co-ordinate, to integrate and to make the courts more user-friendly. Even after 4 years, it is too early to evaluate the legislation but it is a genuine attempt to streamline the law within a framework that tries to balance the often competing interests of the child, the parent and the state, and to provide practical and effective measures.

MAIN PROVISIONS OF THE ACT

Some of the more important aspects of public and private law are dealt with briefly in the space available.

Public law

Part IV of the Act (sections 31–42) deals with the heart of the public law provisions concerning care and supervision. Section 31(2) sets out the threshold conditions, one of which must be proved by the local authority before the court is in a position to consider whether a care or supervision order should be made. A court may only make an order if it is satisfied:

a)   that the child concerned is suffering, or is likely to suffer, significant harm; and
b)   that harm, or likelihood of harm, is attributable to
   i)   the care given to the child, or likely to be given to him if the order were not made, not being what would be reasonable to expect a parent to give to him; or
   ii) the child's being beyond parental control.

Section 31(9) contains important definitions. 'Harm' means ill-treatment or the impairment of health or development. 'Development' means physical, intellectual, emotional, social or behavioural development. 'Health' means physical or mental health; and 'ill-treatment' includes sexual abuse and forms of ill-treatment which are not physical. 'Significant' is not defined and appears, as a result of a lack of reported cases, not to have caused any difficulty in the courts. Section 31(10) states that where the question of whether harm suffered by the child is significant turns on the child's health or development, his health or development shall be compared with that which could reasonably be expected of a similar child.

In *Re M*,[3] the House of Lords, reversing the Court of Appeal, held that 'is suffering' significant harm has to be proved to be occurring at the time when the local authority began the procedure for the protection of the child, provided those arrangements have been continuously in place until the time of the hearing. If the protective arrangements have been terminated, because the child's interests have been otherwise provided for satisfactorily, the test of 'is suffering' will have to be applied at the date of the hearing. The House of Lords has further decided in *Re H*[4] that 'likely' to suffer significant harm means a real possibility, a possibility that cannot sensibly be ignored having regard to the nature and gravity of the feared harm in the particular case. A conclusion that the child is likely to suffer significant harm must be based on facts and not just suspicion.

Part V of the Act (sections 43–52) deals with the emergency protection of children. In particular, child assessment orders and emergency protection orders are provided. A child assessment order[g] may be made by the court, on the application of a local authority or the NSPCC, if it is satisfied that the local authority has reasonable cause to suspect that the child is suffering, or is likely to suffer, significant harm; and an assessment of the state of the child's health or development or the way in which he has been treated, is required to enable the local authority to determine whether or not the child is suffering or is likely to suffer significant harm. Additionally, it has to be proved that it is unlikely that such an assessment will be made, or be satisfactory, in the absence of an order. The assessment may last for a maximum period of 7 days from the date specified in the order.

The emergency protection order,[h] which replaces the place of safety order, may be granted on the application of any person who proves that there is reasonable cause to believe that the child is likely to suffer significant harm if he is not removed to accommodation provided by the applicant or he does not remain in the place in which he is then being accommodated. The order may be made for 8 days and renewed for a further 7.[i] It gives the applicant parental responsibility for the child.

---

3 *Re M* [1994] 2 FLR 577
4 *Re H* [1996] 2 WLR 8

Both provisions expressly provide that a child of sufficient understanding to make an informed decision may refuse to submit to a medical or psychiatric examination or other assessment. This has been said, however, to be subject to the inherent jurisdiction of the High Court.[j]

PRIVATE LAW

The core of the private law provisions are contained in Part II of the Act (sections 8–16). Section 8 orders (residence, contact, prohibited steps and specific issue) replace orders for custody or care and control and related orders. A prohibited steps order means 'an order that no step which could be taken by a parent in meeting his parental responsibility for a child, and which is of a kind specified in the order, shall be taken by any person without the consent of the court'.

A specific issue order means 'an order giving directions for the purpose of determining a specific question which has arisen, or which may arise, in connection with any aspect of parental responsibility for a child'. Applications, for instance, to seek authorization for the sterilisation of a 17-year-old girl or authorization for the use of blood products on a child, against the parents' wishes, can be properly brought for a specific issue order.

The misnamed 'child divorce' cases have been one novel consequence of the statute. With the leave of the court,[k] a child can seek orders relating to his or her residence and contact. A number of unreported cases have each involved a teenage girl who wishes to escape the attentions of a stepfather or a partner of her mother. Solicitors have usually obtained legal aid on behalf of the girl and then sought an order under section 8 in the High Court.

OTHER PROVISIONS

Part III of the Act deals with local authority support for children and families; Part VI with community homes; Part VII with voluntary homes and organisations; Part VIII with registered children's homes; Part IX with private arrangements for fostering children; Part X with childminding and day care for young children and Part XI with the Secretary of State's supervisory functions and responsibilities. Appeals are dealt with in section 94 and the restrictions on the use of wardship in section 100.

ASSESSMENT

The Act has been in force for 4 years. Although it is too early for a proper evaluation, it is quite apparent that the code of law set up has provided greater clarity, certainty and consistency. The interests of children can only be furthered by this much-needed reforming statute.

REFERENCES

a   For a commentary on the Act, see Department of Health 1991/2 The Children
    Act 1989 Guidance and Regulations, volumes 1–10. HMSO, London
b   Cmnd. 62
c   Cmnd. 412
d   See London Borough of Brent 1985 The Jasmine Beckford Report; London
    Borough of Lambeth 1987 The Tyra Henry Report; and London Borough of
    Greenwich 1987 The Kimberley Carlile Report
e   Law Commission Working Papers nos 91; 96; 100; 101; Report no. 100
f   See section 1(2)
g   Section 43
h   Sections 44 and 45
i   But see section 45(2)
j   See sections 43(8) and 44(7); and S. Glamorgan C.C. v B [1993] 1 FLR 574; and
    for further consideration of consent to medical treatment, see Chapter 4 of this
    book
k   See section 10(8)

13. Medical negligence

Ian Wall

An individual who has suffered personal injury as a result of medical intervention will often wish to seek financial compensation. Currently the only way to obtain this redress is by pursuing an action for negligence through the courts.

NEGLIGENCE

Negligence is considered under that part of the civil law which deals with civil wrongs or *torts*. An action in negligence will only succeed when a predetermined legal formula is fulfilled. The elements of this formula are:

1. That there exists between the parties a nexus, or relationship, which gives rise to a *duty of care*.
2. That this duty of care has in some way been broken or *breached* due to the unreasonable acts or omissions of one of the parties, and it is this breach of the duty of care that is the essence of negligence.
3. That in addition the injured party must have suffered *damage, loss* or *injury* of a type that the law recognises.
4. That this damage has been *caused* by the other party.
5. Finally that any action must be brought within a specified time after the injury has occurred (the *limitation period*).

Parties

National Health Service Trusts and Authorities are the usual defendants in medical malpractice suits. They owe a duty of care directly to the patient,[1] and will often be responsible in law for the negligent action of their employees committed in the course of their

---

1 *Cassidy* v *Ministry of Health* [1951] 2KB 343

employment (vicarious liability). As financial compensation is at the heart of an action in negligence, such bodies will possess the necessary financial resources to satisfy any judgment against them.

Duty of care

A duty of care is said to exist when two parties are involved in a close and proximate relationship,[a] where one party can reasonably foresee that by his action he is likely to cause harm to the other party. It is a well established principle of professional relationships that the courts regard doctors, nurses, physiotherapists and pharmacists as owing their patients or clients such a duty of care.

Breach of duty and the standard of care

Once it has been established that a duty exists, the court will examine the conduct of the parties in order to ensure that a minimum standard of competence has been attained. This is the 'standard of care', and in ordinary cases of negligence it is objectively calibrated by reference to what the *reasonable*[b] man would regard as acceptable conduct, and not what the individual concerned thought was reasonable.

NEGLIGENCE IN HEALTHCARE

Healthcare workers, as professionals, will be expected by the courts to exercise care and skill, above and beyond that which the courts would expect of the ordinary reasonable person. The standard governing such professional conduct is stated in *Bolam* v *Friern Hospital Management Committee* [1957][2]:

'The test is the standard of the ordinary skilled man exercising and professing to have a special skill. A man need not possess the highest expert skill at the risk of being found negligent. It is a well established law that it is sufficient if he exercises the ordinary skill of an ordinary man exercising that particular art.'

In assessing therefore whether a practitioner's conduct has fallen below the required standard, the court will have regard to the body of opinion of those practitioners of a similar standing as to

---

2 *Bolam* v *Friern Hospital Management Committee* [1957] 2 All ER 118

whether the actions complained of were in accordance with accepted clinical practice.

It is not enough, however, for the practitioner to attempt to evade liability by calling a number of fellow practitioners to say that what he did, or did not do, was in such accordance.

The court will not accept this body of opinion unquestioningly, but will itself decide whether the complainant has been put at risk by the practice in question, and whether the practice was indeed *reasonable*.[3]

Just as the standard for healthcare professionals is higher than that of the non-qualified, so the standards of specialists are expected to be higher than those of generalists.[4]

The issue of experience came under scrutiny in *Wilsher* v *Essex HA*.[5] Here a senior house officer had inserted an umbilical catheter into a pre-term baby in order to monitor the oxygen concentration in the blood. Unsure as to its position he sought the advice of his registrar, who was of the opinion that the catheter was correctly sited, when in fact it was not. As a consequence the infant received excessive quantities of oxygen which it was later contended caused him to develop blindness. The Court of Appeal concluded that the novice should be judged by the same standards as the experienced practitioner, with no allowance made for lack of training, that is, that the duty should be tailored to the act and not the actor. Junior doctors must therefore exercise skill and care in the decisions they make as to which procedures to undertake unsupervised, and which to defer to more senior colleagues. Because the senior house officer in Wilsher had sought the advice of a more experienced colleague (the registrar) he was able to evade liability.

Specific breaches of duty

The requirement that the professional should exercise reasonable care and skill is in fact a general principle stated in general terms.

In practice the professional will undertake a multiplicity of activities, all with attendant duties. A doctor has a duty to attend and treat his patients; he will not automatically be liable for an

---

3 *Bolitho* v *Hackney* [1993] 4 Med LR 381
4 *Sidaway* v *Governors of Bethlem Royal Hospital and the Maudsley Hospital* [1985] AC 871. Specialists will be expected to attain the standard of those practitioners professing to have that particular skill
5 *Wilsher* v *Essex Area Health Authority* [1986] 3 All ER 801 (CA); [1988] 1 All ER 871 (HL)

incorrect diagnosis, but he will be expected to arrive at the diagnosis with due care and skill, missing only conditions that any other reasonably competent practitioner would also fail to diagnose.

It is the duty of the doctor to keep up with advances in medical practice. He is, however, not required to have an exhaustive knowledge of recent advances and is not under a duty to put into operation all the suggestions of contributors to medical journals, unless they are standard practice.[6]

A doctor has a duty to communicate to his patient any risks (but not all) involved in treatment, to refer to a specialist when appropriate, and to arrange diagnostic tests when appropriate. In private medicine a practitioner may also be liable to his patient in contract,[7] for breach of an *implied* contractual term to provide his services with due skill and care. In rare circumstances the practitioner has even been regarded as having guaranteed that his treatment would succeed.

Damage

Proof that *damage*, loss or injury has occurred is vital in cases of negligence, as the law does not hold actionable so-called 'negligence in the air'. Thus no matter how careless or inadvertent a course of action is, provided it does not cause any injury, there is no liability. The damage, furthermore, must be of a type that the court recognises as legally actionable. For example the psychological sequelae, such as anxiety and distress, resulting from a negligent act will only warrant compensation if they amount to a recognised psychiatric condition.[8]

Causation

Causation is the connection between the negligent act and the damage or injury suffered. In order to succeed on the issue of factual causation the plaintiff[c] has to show that '*but for the defendant's fault, on the balance of probability, the injury complained of (or the 'gist' of the damage) would not have occurred*'.[d]

In *Barnett* v *Chelsea and Kensington Hospital Management Committee*[9] the defendant's employee, a doctor, in breach of his

---

6 *Crawford* v *Board of Governors of Charing Cross Hospital, The Times,* 8 December 1953
7 *Thake* v *Maurice* [1986] 1 All ER 499
8 *McLoughlin* v *O'Brian* [1982] 2 All ER 298
9 *Barnett* v *Chelsea and Kensington Hospital Management Committee* [1969] 1 QB 428

duty had declined to see a patient who, unbeknown to all, had been the victim of a poisoner. In the civil action following the patient's death, the court found that by the time he arrived at the hospital his fate was sealed. The plaintiff was therefore unable to satisfy the 'but for' test, because notwithstanding the defendant's negligence, the patient would have perished anyway.

The 'balance of probability' limb is the degree of cogency or persuasiveness required of the plaintiff's evidence (evidential standard of proof) on the factual issues. This means that the plaintiff, in order to discharge the burden of proving his case, has to adduce sufficient factual evidence to persuade the court that it was more probable than not (i.e. greater than 50%) that the defendant's actions had caused his injury.[e]

In simple cases, where there is clear medical and scientific evidence, the issue of causation poses little practical or conceptual difficulty. Medical interactions are, however, often complex. Factual scientific evidence may suggest an association between insult and injury, but may not be cogent enough to support a causative link. Furthermore there is often a lack of concrete statistical material to introduce into the balance of probability scales. Under these circumstances therefore a plaintiff will be doomed to fail on the causation issue. In order to alleviate the potential unfairness of this situation for plaintiffs, the courts under certain circumstances will bridge this 'evidential gap' by *inferring* causation. In *McGhee* v *NCB* [1972][10] a kiln worker, who was in the ordinary course of his work exposed to brick dust (the 'innocent' dust), claimed that as a result of the defendant employer's breach of duty in failing to provide washing facilities, he was subject to a prolonged exposure to the brick dust (the 'guilty' dust) by being forced to cycle home with it on his skin. It could not be shown, as a matter of scientific fact, that it was the prolongation of exposure that had caused the dermatitis, and thus the 'but for' test was not satisfied. The courts reasoned that in the absence of definitive proof, it was a legitimate inference of fact that the defendant's negligence had materially contributed to or increased the *risk* of the injury occurring.

In *Wilsher* the 'but for' test foundered because excess oxygen was but one of several factors present which may have led to the blindness, the others not being the result of the defendant's breach of duty. The House of Lords would not extend the inferential reasoning of *McGhee*, which allowed them to separate guilty and innocent

---

10 *McGhee* v *NCB* [1972] All ER 1008

components of one possible causative agent (brick dust), into situations where there were a number (excess oxygen, prematurity, brain haemorrhages). The House of Lords stated that the defendant's administration of excessive oxygen 'provided no evidence and raised no presumption that it was this insult rather than the several others present which had caused the defendant's blindness'.

Loss of a chance

The 'but for' test also has the disadvantage of being an 'all or nothing' test, so that provided the defendant does not create a risk greater than the background risk he will not be liable. Attempts by plaintiffs to get around this problem by formulating the gist of the damage into the loss of a chance have met with limited success.[11]

Special groups

The scope of the doctor's duty of care can extend beyond his immediate patients, to others. This is because they form a group of individuals who may also reasonably be contemplated as sustaining injury as a result of his actions. Examples include the common law duty to a child born disabled as a result of negligent treatment of the mother during her pregnancy,[f] and to other road users when assessing an individual's fitness to drive.

Quantum

Quantum, or 'damages', is the pecuniary measure of injuries suffered. The general aim of damages in tort is to put the injured party, so far as is possible, into the position he would have been in if he had not been injured. As such the injured party must be compensated for the injury itself, and its effects on him financially and emotionally.

There are two broad categories, or heads, of damages, namely special damages and general damages, and a claim would ordinarily include both. Special damages represent the actual pecuniary loss between the time the injury was sustained and the trial, and as such are financially quantifiable. Claimable under this head of damage are items such as the cost of purchase of special equipment or appliances (such as wheelchairs), medical expenses, the cost of

---

11 *Hotson* v *East Berkshire Area Health Authority* [1987] 1 All ER 210 (CA) where the
    argument succeeded and [1987] 2 All ER 909 (HL) where it failed and the Court
    of Appeal's ruling was overturned

nursing care, and most importantly the loss of earnings during that period.

General damages essentially represent the compensation for the plaintiff's *future* financial loss, and the loss due to the injuries he has suffered. There are six heads of damage:

1. pain and suffering resulting from the injury
2. loss of amenity or reduced enjoyment of life
3. future loss of earnings
4. loss of earning capacity
5. loss of pension rights, and
6. future expenses.

If the injured party dies as a result of negligence then their estate can continue the action with the executor(s) as the plaintiff.[g]

Limitation period

There is often a temporal delay between a negligent act and the resulting damage and sometimes, though the injury is immediately manifest, it is not evident that it has been caused by the defendant's negligence. To allow the spectre of litigation to hover indefinitely may cause undue hardship, if not just for the practical difficulties involved in adducing and interpreting stale evidence. The Limitation Act 1980 (s11) imposes a time limit of 3 years on litigants bringing an action for negligence resulting in personal injury, and claims outside this period will be barred. The clock starts to run from the date at which the action accrued, or alternatively the time when the plaintiff realised that his injury was significant and was a result of a negligent action by the defendant whom he is able to identify (s14).

The court maintains a jurisdiction to override the limitation provisions in exceptional cases if, having regard to all the circumstances of the case, neither party would be prejudiced by allowing the action to proceed out of time. Under s33 the court will look at such matters as the length and reason for the delay, and the conduct of both parties. If at the time of the injury a person is under 18 years of age, then the limitation period does not begin (i.e. the cause of action does not accrue) until they attain majority, or if mentally ill until they recover (s28).

Involuntary manslaughter

There has been an increased willingness by the authorities to undertake the criminal prosecution of doctors whose patients die as a result of their mistakes. In *R* v *Adamoko* [1991][12] the Court of Appeal[h] stated that in cases where there is a breach of duty causing death, a jury should only convict when it regarded the conduct as being 'grossly negligent'[i]. The test advanced in the Court of Appeal would permit individual circumstances, excuses and explanations to be advanced by way of mitigating criminal liability.

CONCLUSION

Civil litigation can be time-consuming, expensive and beset with evidential obstacles. Success in a civil action for negligence will result in finding the professional concerned at fault, when perhaps the principal motivational force for bringing an action was not to punish but to obtain an explanation for what had gone wrong or to establish future financial support. Furthermore the issue of causation will often prove insurmountable. Other jurisdictions, such as New Zealand and Sweden, have introduced 'no fault' compensation for victims of medical accidents where proof of negligence is not required. Such schemes have their own problems, and their long-term economic viability is questionable. In the UK, the likely effects of the proposed introduction of a streamlining of litigation and a contingent fees system have yet to be fully assessed.

REFERENCES

a   This relationship is often called the 'neighbour' principle and was initially formulated by Lord Atkin in *Donoghue* v *Stevenson* [1932] AC 562, and followed and extended as a general principle in later cases, e.g. *Home Office* v *Dorset Yacht Co Ltd*. [1970] AC 1004. Recent trends have seen a retreat from this broad principle
b   The reasonable man is an ubiquitous legal fiction often referred to as the man on the Clapham Omnibus. He is the 'ordinary man' whose fictional perspective acts as an objective fixed point when judging conduct, thereby providing some consistency between cases by eliminating subjective personal characteristics, such as experience, education or mental capacity
c   The plaintiff or patient will bear the burden of proving the case, under the principle 'he who asserts must prove'
d   This is the general rule on the standard of proof in all civil cases.
    Miller v *Minister of Pensions* [1947] 2 All ER 372
e   This legal concept is far removed from the certainties that scientists search for to prove cause and effect (e.g. the attempts to link leukaemia to radiation)

---

12   *R* v *Adamoko* [1991] 2 Med LR 277

f   There is also a statutory duty under the Congenital Disabilities (Civil Liability) Act 1976, for babies born prior to 1976
g   Law Reform (Miscellaneous Provisions) Act 1934
h   The Appeal in *Adamoko* in fact concerned two cases, *R* v *Prentice and Sullman* where two junior doctors stood accused of manslaughter after wrongly administering a cytotoxic drug into the spine of a patient who subsequently died, and *R* v *Adamoko* where a patient died when an anaesthetist had failed to notice that an oxygen tube had become disconnected
i   Barker I 1993 Manslaughter conviction quashed. Journal of the Medical Defence Union 3: 52

FURTHER READING

Powers M, Harris N 1994 Medical negligence, 2nd edn. Butterworths, London (*a legal practitioner's book*)
Kemp D (ed) 1992 Kemp and Kemp: The quantum of damages. Sweet and Maxwell, London (*a loose-leaf guide to quanta based on judicial awards for particular injuries*)

14. The Medicines Act and product liability

Ivor Harrison

INTRODUCTION

The Medicines Act 1968 was passed in the aftermath of the Thalidomide disaster.[a] It was intended to ensure that medicines were marketed only after their quality, safety and efficacy had been assessed by independent experts and licensed by the government. The Act controlled all aspects of the development, manufacture, packaging and labelling, distribution and advertising of medicines both for human and for animal use. The Act provided a basic structure of controls and left the detail to be made by means of statutory instruments (orders and regulations), over 150 of which have subsequently been made by the Ministers. At the centre of the controls is a licensing system under which each product must be the subject of a product licence (s7(2)). It must be manufactured and packed as specified in that licence by someone holding an appropriate manufacturer's licence (s8(2)), be dealt with by licensed wholesalers (s8(3)) and then distributed to consumers usually via pharmacists or practitioners (s52). Fees are charged for the licences (Medicines Act 1971) and the scales of fees are laid down in Regulations (SI 1991 No. 1474 as amended). The fee income is designed to meet the costs incurred in administering the Act. Breach of a term or condition of a licence can lead to powerful sanctions such as suspension or revocation of the licence (s28(2)).

All licences contain 'standard provisions' (s47) which apply to the licence holder. Among these is the requirement to notify the licensing authority of any change to his name and address, of any change that he intends to make to the specifications of the product, its method or place of manufacture, packaging or labelling. He must also inform the authority of any information he receives that casts doubt on the continued validity of the data supplied in the application for a product licence. For further details see The

Medicines (Standard Provisions for Licences and Certificates) Regulations 1971 (SI 1971 No. 972 and amendments).

Definition of 'medicinal product'

A medicinal product is defined as 'any substance or article (not being an instrument, apparatus or appliance) which is manufactured, sold, supplied, imported or exported for use wholly or mainly in either or both of the following ways . . .

a. use by being administered to one or more human beings or animals for a medicinal purpose;
b. use (in a pharmacy, or by a practitioner or herbalist) as an ingredient in the preparation of a substance . . . to be administered . . . for a medicinal purpose (s130(1)).

'Medicinal purpose' means any one or more of the following purposes:

a. treating or preventing disease
b. diagnosing disease or ascertaining the existence, degree or extent of a physiological condition
c. contraception
d. inducing anaesthesia
e. otherwise preventing or interfering with the normal operation of a physiological function, whether permanently or temporarily, and whether by way of terminating, reducing or postponing, or increasing or accelerating, the operation of that function or in any other way. (s130(2)).

There are ministerial powers to make Orders imposing similar controls over substances and articles which fall outside the above definitions (s104; s105) or to exempt products from some or all of the controls (s130(5)).

Borderline substances

The definitions cited above encompass various products which are on the borderline between medicines and foods, cosmetics or devices. The issue is normally resolved by examining the way in which the product is to be sold or promoted. If medicinal claims are made, then it is a medicine. The European Court of Justice has given several important decisions relating to these borderline products (see *van Bennekom* ECJ;[1] *Delattre* ECJ).[2]

---

1 *van Bennekom* ECJ Case 227/82 [1983] ECR 3883
2 *Delattre* ECJ Case C-369/88

Data required in an application for a Product Licence

An enormous amount of scientific effort is expended during the development of a new drug substance. In the search for a new chemical having therapeutic potential, 5000–10 000 new substances will be synthesised and screened. Those showing promise are subjected to detailed chemical and toxicological study. The chemical studies are performed to identify and characterise the substance, to find the best synthetic routes and to identify the by-products which occur during synthesis. It is also necessary to develop analytical methods capable of detecting the substance and measuring precisely how much of it is present in a number of different situations, such as its concentration in blood, tissue fluids, urine, faeces.

The toxicological studies are necessary to determine whether the substance causes serious damage to the vital organs of laboratory animals and to study the ways in which they metabolise the drug. After about 4 years' work, all but about 10 substances will have been rejected because they had no worthwhile activity, were too toxic or perhaps too unstable. The remaining substances are then administered to a few human volunteers in order to determine which of the experimental animals most closely resembles the human in terms of metabolising the drug. This also ensures that the substance still has a worthwhile therapeutic activity. Usually, about half of the remaining drug candidates are rejected at this stage. The rest are subjected to clinical trial, that is, administered to a small number of patients suffering from one of the conditions for which it is indicated that the drug will prove efficacious.

Originally scientists decided what methods, tests and criteria to use to satisfy themselves as to the value of the new substance. Full details of all the tests and the results obtained over the development period were written and sent to the Medicines Control Agency (MCA) (formerly the Medicines Division) for assessment. Preliminary data also had to be supplied when application was made for the product to be put to clinical trial. The Act required the sponsor of a trial to hold either a Clinical Trial Certificate (CTC) (s31) or a Clinical Trial Exemption Certificate (CTX) (SI 1981 No. 164) for each trial.

As part of the harmonisation process for licensing medicines within the European Union, numerous criteria and guidelines have been developed. Although the regulatory bodies insist that many are merely 'guidelines', not tramlines, any failure to adhere to them must be explained. In 1980, the OECD published a document entitled Principles of Good Laboratory Practice (GLP)[b] to ensure that data generated in laboratory tests were of the highest quality. Moreover, compliance with the Principles enabled both the tests and the assessment of their results to be performed uniformly in different countries. The European Directives on pharmaceuticals state that all the development work on new drugs must be done to GLP standards. Similar guidelines are being produced to ensure that clinical trials are likewise carried out in a way comparable with tests (Good Clinical Practice)[c] These guidelines are collected together and published periodically in the series 'The Rules Governing Medicinal Products in the European Community'.[d]

Assessment of the data

To obtain a product licence, the applicant must send to the licensing authority full details of the method of manufacture and of the tests performed on the product (and on its ingredients) which prove that it is safe, of good quality and efficacious. In the case of a product containing a new active substance, this work will typically take 10–12 years to complete and currently cost about £200 million. This evidence will be examined by the Committee on Safety of Medicines (CSM) if for human use. Products for animal use are examined by the Veterinary Products Committee (VPC). Where a product consists of substances of known efficacy, safety and quality the application is much smaller in volume and is assessed by the professional staff of the Medicines Control Agency (MCA).

Expert committees

Expert committees were created to advise the 'Licensing Authority' (i.e. the Ministers) on the safety, quality and efficacy of medicines (s4). The CSM (SI 1970 No. 1257) and VPC (SI 1970 No. 1304) are two such bodies. The Medicines Commission has a supervisory role over the committees and also has appellate functions which unsuccessful applicants can invoke if desired (s2; s3; sched.1). The members of the expert committees (and of the Commission) are appointed by the Ministers and are persons having expertise in various fields of medical, pharmaceutical and related sciences. They come largely from academic bodies and the pharmaceutical industry. In order to ensure the impartiality of their advice, they are required to register their shareholdings in pharmaceutical companies, and any consultancies, research grants, etc., that they hold. The CSM is also responsible for the collection and assessment of reports of adverse reactions to all medicines, and for the publication of warnings when necessary.

Legal liability of the licensing authority and of its advisors

Some years ago the Opren Action Group commenced an action against the manufacturers of the product and also against the licensing authority and the CSM.[3] The case was settled out of court by the manufacturer so judicial opinion on the liability of the last named defendants was not forthcoming. The validity of any decision of the licensing authority in relation to a licensing matter shall not be questioned in any legal proceedings except on the grounds that either it was *ultra vires* or that the Authority had failed to comply with any requirement of the Act or of any regulations made under it (s107). However, the Act states that neither the Commission nor any expert committee 'shall be taken to be the servant or agent of the Crown or to enjoy any status or immunity of the Crown' (sched. 1 para. 7). Arising out of this, the Department of Health gave undertakings to members of the CSM (and the other expert committees) that the Department would pay the legal costs of any member personally subject to any action arising out of the business of the committee.[e]

Manufacturing methods and controls

Every manufacturer of a medicine has to be licensed with the Medicines Control Agency (s8). An applicant for a manufacturer's licence must show that his premises, equipment and staff are such that the products made will meet the highest standards (SI 1971 No. 973 as amended). In addition, he must employ as 'qualified person' someone having the necessary qualifications and experience to ensure that the processes are carried out to specification and that every batch of every product has met the quality assurance criteria specified in the relevant product licence. Manufacturing premises are inspected regularly and inspectors are entitled to inspect products, processes and plant and to take samples and make copies of documents. In this context, 'manufacture' includes 'assembly', that is, packaging and labelling of

---

3 *Nash* v *Eli Lilly* [1991] 2 Med LR 169

products made by someone else. Pharmacists in retail pharmacies and hospitals, practitioners and herbalists are exempt from these provisions when they make preparations for their own patients (s9; s10; s12).

Wholesale dealers

Wholesale dealers require a licence which is only granted to persons who have the appropriate facilities for the correct storage of medicines. Dealers have to maintain records (including batch numbers) of goods inward and outward to facilitate recall of products if necessary.

Packaging and labelling

To maintain the quality of a product it must be packed in a container to protect it from air, from light and from moisture, all of which can have a deleterious effect upon the product's quality, safety and efficacy. It may be necessary to store the product within a specified temperature range, and to facilitate this, the container and all outer packagings must be clearly labelled to that effect and must carry the batch number and expiry date.

Labelling is also very important in promoting the safety and efficacy of the product. The label should identify the product, each of its active ingredients and their amounts, the optimum dosage for each of the licensed indications, any precautions to be taken and any major side-effects such as interactions with common foods or other drugs and potential for causing drowsiness. Its expiry date is also important, as is the batch number which facilitates recall if faults subsequently become apparent in the product. The law also requires various other details to be included on the label such as the product licence number, the manufacturer's licence number and the legal class of the product. The pharmaceutical company often has difficulty in including all of this information legibly on labels for small containers. Very detailed requirements were imposed by the Medicines (Labelling) Regulations 1976 which have been amended 12 times to date. The most recent amendments (SI 1992 No. 3273), implement changes necessary to conform to Directive 92/26/EEC. The main changes include:

- the need to use the 'common name', that is, the International Non-Proprietary Name for the active ingredient(s) whereas formerly a pharmacopoeial name could be used
- the need to include a list of those excipients (components forming the basis of the remainder of the ingredients) used which are known to have a recognised action or effect
- a requirement to list ALL excipients in injections, eye preparations and topicals
- a need to include any requirements of the product licence applicable to the disposal of unused product.

It is possible that guidelines as to the excipients mentioned in (b) above will be issued in future. In the meantime, the MCA have issued a suggested list.[f]

Leaflets

Unlike many other countries in which original pack dispensing is the norm, in the United Kingdom little use was made of leaflets. However, leaflets are now obligatory unless all of the information required to be given in a leaflet is printed and visible on the label. The legal requirements are given in the Leaflets Regulations 1992 No. 3274. The leaflets must not be promotional. The leaflet must:

- identify the product, state names and amounts of all active ingredients and the names of all excipients, the pharmaceutical form and contents by weight, volume or number of doses, the pharmaco-therapeutic group (in easily understood terms) and the name and address of the licence holder
- state its therapeutic indications
- list information which is necessary before taking the product including contraindications, precautions, interactions and special warnings
- include instructions for the proper use of the product including dosage, method and if necessary route of administration, frequency of administration, and if appropriate duration of treatment, action in case of overdosage, what to do if a dose is missed
- include description of undesirable effects and if necessary of action to be taken, together with an express invitation to inform the doctor or pharmacist of any effect not mentioned in the leaflet

- include a reference to the expiry date on the label and a warning against using it after the date, any special storage conditions and if necessary a warning against certain visible signs of deterioration
- give the date of last revision of leaflet.

Controls over distribution

The Medicines Act restricted the sale of medicines to pharmacies. For the convenience of the public an exception was made for those products specified in the General Sale List (GSL) (s51) as being sufficiently safe to be sold without the supervision of a pharmacist. The GSL products must have been packed and labelled for sale at premises other than those from which they are retailed, and must be sold in unopened containers (s53).

The majority of other medicines may only be supplied to the public on the prescription of a medical, dental or veterinary practitioner — prescription only medicines (POM).

Quality

Manufacturers of medicines take considerable care to ensure the quality of their products (see above). However, the quality of a product can be seriously impaired by faulty storage or by accidental or deliberate contamination. The Act makes it an offence to adulterate any medicinal product or to possess, offer or expose for sale or supply a product which has been adulterated (s63). Similarly, it is an offence to sell to the prejudice of the purchaser a product not of the nature or quality demanded (s64). Where a product is demanded (either by a purchaser or a prescriber) by reference to a name which is used at the head of a monograph in an official book of standards (such as a pharmacopoeia), a product which complies with all the specifications of that monograph must be supplied (s65). These provisions of the Act are enforced by inspectors who make test purchases at shops, including pharmacies. There is no provision, however, for the quality of medicines dispensed by doctors, dentists or veterinarians or from hospitals to be subject to test.

Controls over promotion of sales

The Act defined 'advertisement' in very broad terms and distinguished it from 'representations' (spoken words) (s92(1), (5)).

Offences relating either to advertisements or representations can only be committed by 'commercially interested parties', that is, persons who have some financial interest in selling the product such as the product licence holder, a wholesaler or a retailer (s92(4)). It is an offence for anyone other than the product licence holder to issue an advertisement relating to a product (s94). It is also an offence to issue an advertisement or a representation which is false or misleading (s93(1), (3)), or one containing an unauthorised recommendation (that is, for a purpose not specified in the product licence) (s93(2), (4), (10)).

Regulations have been made to specify the information that must be included in advertisements sent or directed to medical and dental practitioners. A licensed product cannot be promoted to practitioners until a data sheet has been issued for that product. This must contain all of the information specified in the Data Sheet Regulations and include the clinical indications for which it is licensed. Under regulations (SI 1994 No. 1932) made to implement Directive 92/28, in future all advertisements directed to health professionals will have to contain 'essential information compatible with the summary of product characteristics'. The term 'essential information' is not defined in the Directive but Schedule 2 to the Regulations lists the UK requirements. They closely resemble the data sheet. The same regulations require licence holders to set up a scientific service to collect and collate information from all sources relating to that product. In addition they shall provide proper training for sales representatives and provide them with complete and precise information about the holder's products. The licence holder must comply immediately and fully with any decision of the licensing authority relating to an advertisement issued by him.

Special requirements apply to reference advertisements, abbreviated advertisements (those loosely inserted in medical journals and not exceeding 420 square centimetres in area) and trade advertisements.

A separate set of regulations (SI 1978 No.41) control advertisements directed to the public. It is an offence to advertise to the public a product for human use which is either a Prescription Only Medicine or is indicated for the treatment or prevention of one of the diseases specified in schedule 1 or for most dysfunctions of the body. In summary, only remedies for trivial, self-limiting conditions can be advertised to the public.

Prosecutions

There have been three prosecutions for advertising offences. The first involved a person who ran a mail-order business in sex aids who was convicted of three charges of advertising them in terms which contravened the prohibition on 'enhancement of sexual potency or libido'.[4] The second involved the sale of first aid kits for travellers overseas which contained some POMs together with indications for their use.[5] The third case involved the pharmaceutical company Roussel and its Medical Director who were each convicted of issuing false or misleading advertisements (the same advertisement in five issues of the British Medical Journal).[6]

Codes of Practice

In addition to the law, there are Codes of Practice which control advertisements for medicines in the UK. These Codes are recognised by the law and are compatible with it. The Association of British Pharmaceutical Industry has a Code which is administered by the Prescription Medicines Code of Practice Authority. This Authority provides advice and guidance on the Code and routinely scrutinises journal advertising. There is a Code of Practice Panel to consider complaints about advertisements, and also an Appeal Board chaired by an independent, legally qualified chairman.

The Proprietary Association of Great Britain (PAGB) set up its Code in 1936 and has kept it up to date ever since.[g] The Code requires the manufacturers of 'patent' medicines to submit drafts of advertisements for clearance before they are issued. This Code is recognised by the Advertising Standards Authority, complies with its rules and is subject to its sanctions.

Liability

The Medicines Acts aimed to prevent injury to consumers of medicinal products rather than to compensate them for such injuries. Medicines are inherently dangerous, so inevitably someone will suffer damage after consuming a medicine. The damage may result from an idiosyncratic reaction on the part of the patient and not be due to any defect in the product. The damage may vary in serious-

---

4 Medicines Act Information Letter 1982 no 33 Item 17a. Medicines Division, London
5 East Kent Mercury 23 Jan 86 (reporting prosecution for advertising offences)
6 *R* v *Roussel Laboratories Ltd* [1989] 88 Cr. App. R 140

ness from transient symptoms such as headache, itching or diarrhoea to more serious effects such as blood dyscrasias or loss of vision and even to death. At the other extreme, a manufacturing error could kill or injure the majority of persons exposed to the product. The quality assurance procedures used by manufacturers should detect such errors long before the product is released for sale but if they failed, the manufacturer would clearly be liable. The problems really arise where the product is not defective but causes unforeseen damage to a (generally) small proportion of consumers.

The law of contract and also the Sale of Goods Act 1979 provide remedies for purchasers of products which are not of merchantable quality or are unfit for the purpose, and thereby injure the purchaser. Thus a person who is injured by a defective medicine which he bought can sue the supplier (not necessarily the manufacturer) for damages. If the product had been bought by a third party, the injured person could sue in tort[7] but would have to prove that the manufacturer had been negligent. Similarly, patients who suffer harm from medicines supplied under the National Health Service are not 'purchasers'[8] and would therefore have to sue in tort. To succeed in such an action, the plaintiff would have to prove that:-
a. he had suffered damage (physical, mental or economic)
b. the damage was the result of an act or omission on the part of the manufacturer
c. a competent manufacturer would have foreseen the damage and taken steps to avoid the mistake.

In practice, it is frequently difficult to prove that the damage did result from negligence on the part of the manufacturer. For example, before Thalidomide was marketed, there were no tests for teratogenicity of drugs. The situation was changed by the Directive on Product Liability (85/374/EEC) which was implemented in the UK by the Consumer Protection Act 1987. The plaintiff no longer has to prove negligence on the part of the defendant, but has to show:

a.   that the product had a defect
b.   that he suffered damage caused by that defect
c.   that the defendant was the 'producer' of the product.

The 'producer' might be the actual manufacturer, the person who imported it into the European Union, or the person who had his

---

7 *Donoghue* v *Stevenson* [1932] AC 562. The leading case, establishing many
   principles fundamental to the law of negligence, including duty of care
8 *Pfizer Corporation* v *Ministry of Health* 1 All ER 1965, 450–479

name on the product as the 'producer'. In the context of this Act, 'defective' is closely related to safety and in deciding whether a product is or is not defective the manner and purposes for which the product was marketed and any instructions or warnings which are given with it are relevant. Also of importance is what may reasonably be expected of it: how and why the product might be used. The time when the product was made may also be important because standards of safety are constantly improving.

Six defences are provided by the Act (s4) but the most important to medicines are:

i.   'That the defect is attributable to compliance with any requirement imposed by or under any enactment or with a Community obligation' (s4(a)). This does not mean that products which have been licensed by the government are certified as free from defects.

ii.   'That the state of scientific and technical knowledge at the relevant time was not such that the producer of products of the same description as the product in question might be expected to have discovered the defect if it had existed in his products while they were under his control' (s4(e)). This is the 'development risk' defence. In essence it means that the producer can escape liability for a defect which was not apparent when the article was made because no suitable tests for the defect existed at the time. Thus, the Act would not have helped the victims of Thalidomide. Although the Directive permitted national governments to incorporate this defence into their laws, consumer groups and others have protested at its inclusion.

European Community law

There is a corresponding body of European Community law, and the European Medicines Evaluation Agency has been created to issue marketing authorisations having effect in every Member State. This will clearly mean a considerable saving of effort for the pharmaceutical industry because it will no longer be necessary to obtain authorisations from each country.

REFERENCES

a   Forthcoming legislation on the Safety, Quality and Description of Drugs and Medicines Cmnd 3395 September 1967

b   Organisation for Economic Cooperation and Development (OECD) 1980 Principles of good laboratory practice (GLP). OECD

c   European Community 1991 Principles of good clinical practice. Directive 91/507/EEC, Luxembourg

d   European Community 1989–1991 Rules governing medicinal products in the European Community, L-2985, Luxembourg:
1991 Vol. I: The rules governing medicinal products for human use in the European Community, revised edn.
1989 Vol. II: Notice to applicants for marketing authorizations for medicinal products for human use in the Member States of the European Community
1989 Vol. III: Guidelines on the quality, safety and efficacy of medicinal products for human use
Addenda to Vol III: 1990; 1992
1989 Vol. IV: Guide to good manufacturing practice for medicinal products

e   Medicines Control Agency 1992 Annual Report 1991–1992: 25. Medicines Control Agency, London

f   Medicines Control Agency 1993 Guidance for the pharmaceutical industry on the labelling and leaflets regulations, Appendix 3. Medicines Control Agency, London

g   Proprietary Association of Great Britain 1986 Code of Standards of Advertising Practice 1936–1986

15. HIV, AIDS and the law

John Skone

INTRODUCTION

The first clinical description of Acquired Immunodeficiency Syndrome (AIDS) in the United States was given in the Morbidity and Mortality Weekly Report of the centers for Disease Control in 1981.[a, b] Editorial notes postulated an association between some aspect of homosexual lifestyle or disease acquired through sexual contact and alerted physicians to Kaposi's sarcoma (KS), *pneumocystis carinii* pneumonia (PCP) and other opportunistic infections associated with immunosuppression in homosexual men.

The Human Immunodeficiency Virus (HIV) was discovered in 1983 and it is now known that the virus is transmitted in three ways:

- unprotected homo- or heterosexual intercourse
- blood to blood contact (as in haemophiliacs, needle-stick occupational injury, blood transfusions, injecting drug users)
- transmission by an infected mother to her baby during pregnancy, birth or breast feeding.

HIV INFECTION AND AIDS IN THE UNITED KINGDOM

The first case of AIDS was reported in 1982. Clinicians in England and Wales are encouraged to send details in confidence to the Director of the Communicable Disease Surveillance Centre (CDSC) at Colindale and in Scotland to the Scottish Centre for Infection and Environmental Health (SCIEH) at Ruchill Hospital, Glasgow. By 31 December 1994, a total of 10 304 reports of AIDS (9414 male and 890 female) had been received, of whom 7019 (68%) were known to have died.

A cumulative total of 23 104 HIV-1 infections were reported since testing began in 1984. Evidence from unlinked anonymous prevalence monitoring indicates that just under half of actual HIV infections are recognised.

The proportion of AIDS cases attributed to sexual intercourse between men ranged from 43% in Scotland to 80% in the four Thames regions. The proportion attributed to injecting drug use was highest in Scotland (36%) compared with 3% in the four Thames regions.

By 31 October 1995, 232 AIDS cases had been reported in the UK in children aged less than 15 years, and 124 were known to have died. Those infected perinatally totalled 181 and 51 were infected following treatment with contaminated blood or blood factor.[c, d]

In 1993 it was estimated that 85–88% of all AIDS cases were being reported in this voluntary surveillance scheme.[e]

The Legal framework in the United Kingdom

Under the National Health Service (Venereal Diseases) Regulations 1974, the identity of persons examined or treated for any sexually transmitted disease can be disclosed only in exceptional circumstances. In the case of X v Y,[1] the court banned a newspaper from using information wrongly extracted from the confidential notes of two medical practitioners with AIDS. It was held that public interests were substantially outweighed when measured against loyalty and confidentiality both generally and in relation to AIDS patients' hospital records.[f]

Consolidating legislation in the Public Health (Control of Disease) Act 1984 is extended by the Public Health (Infectious Diseases) Regulations 1985 to include AIDS. They do not make AIDS a notifiable disease but they apply sections 35 (medical examination), 37 (removal to hospital), 38 (detention in hospital), 43 (restrictions on removal of the body of a person dying in hospital) and 44 (isolation of the body of a person dying outside hospital) to the condition.

Sections 35, 37 and 38 can be activated by order of a single Justice of the Peace (who may make an order, if necessary, *ex parte*). Compulsory medical examination can be ordered only if the magistrate is satisfied, on a written certificate of a medical practitioner nominated by the local authority, that there is reason to believe that a person is suffering from a notifiable disease or is carrying an

---

1 X (Health Authority) v Y [1988] 2 All ER 648

organism capable of carrying it and that it is in the interests of the patient, the family or the public. No order can be made without the consent of a registered medical practitioner treating the patient.

Section 35 orders can be supplemented by orders under section 61 of the Act, in which magistrates can issue warrants to support the entry, if necessary by force, of an authorised officer. Under section 15 wilful neglect or refusal to obey or obstruction in the execution of the Regulations may be punished by a fine, and in the case of a continuing offence by a further fine of up to £50 a day. Section 37 allows a local authority to apply to a magistrate for the removal to hospital of a patient suffering from AIDS. Section 38, relating to detention in hospital, has been modified by Regulation 3 of the 1985 legislation to apply to AIDS.

Because of the small risk of spread of infection, compulsory action is rarely contemplated unless the risks increase, for example haemorrhage, uncontrolled infective diarrhoea and drug-resistant pulmonary or disseminated tuberculosis.

Appeals can be made against orders under sections 35, 37 and 38 initially to the Crown Court. Judicial review would also be available to challenge procedural errors or matters of jurisdiction.

On 14 September 1985 magistrates in Manchester, UK ordered, under Section 38, the detention for three weeks in Monsall Hospital of a 25-year-old man with AIDS. The City Council Medical Officer for Environmental Health said that the patient was 'bleeding copiously and trying to discharge himself'. At appeal in the Crown Court, Counsel for the City said that the man's condition had improved substantially and continued detention was no longer sought. Mr Justice Russell allowed the appeal, but said that in view of the medical evidence the original order was proper. The patient was now said to be willing to remain in hospital. The appeal was uncontested and no case-law was created.[g]

Where a person dies of AIDS in hospital, a proper officer of the local authority (nowadays usually the consultant in Communicable Disease Control) can certify under section 43 that it is desirable, in order to prevent the spread of infection, that the body should not be removed except for transfer to a mortuary or to be cremated or buried; 69% of all bodies are cremated. Provided that the Medical Referee, approved by the Secretary of State for the Home Department, is satisfied that the cause of death has been definitely ascertained, transfer and cremation can take place. Disregard of a certificate is a criminal offence, punishable by a fine.

The AIDS Control Act 1987

This Act came into force on 15 May 1987 and has been amended to take account of administrative changes embodied into the National Health Service and Community Care Act 1990.

The Act provides for the collection and reporting of statistics relating to HIV infection and AIDS and the availability of facilities and staff for testing, consulting, treatment and other measures, in particular health education, designed to prevent the spread of HIV infection. Annual Reports are made to the Regional Health Authority by the District Health Authority, and to the Secretary of State by:

- each regional office in England of the Department of Health's NHS Management Executive; these offices replaced Regional Health Authorities in England
- each District Health Authority in Wales
- each Health Board in Scotland
- each NHS Trust.

The Reports are published.

Regional Health Authorities in England have now been replaced by Regional offices of the Department of Health NHS Management Executive.

Section 23 prevents the sale, supply or administration of any equipment or reagents to detect HIV antibodies (test kits) in centres without medical supervision and no certainty of competent pre- and post-test counselling.

AIDS and blood products

Evidence that AIDS could be contracted from contaminated blood products and particularly from the Factor VIII clotting agent used for treating haemophiliacs was available in late 1982. By mid 1983, high risk blood donors had been identified by research programmes in the field and a system of screening was introduced on a voluntary and self-regulating basis in some countries. Factor VIII was mainly imported into the UK from the USA, and was not universally treated until the end of 1984. The test for HIV antibodies (the 'ELISA' test) became available during 1985. The treatment of existing NHS concentrate started in early 1985 and the new heat-treated product was available from October 1985.

In November 1987 the Government set up a £10 million trust fund for affected haemophiliacs and their families, to make *ex gratia* payments (an average of less than £8500 per family) and not as compensation. In July 1989 the Lord Chief Justice assigned to Mr Justice Ognall the cases of several patients with haemophilia and HIV infection and their families who were suing, or proposed to sue, the Government and Health Authorities, with the intention of coordination along the lines of the 'Opren' litigation[2] referred to in Chapter 14.

On 11 December 1990 it was announced that agreement had been reached between lawyers for the plaintiffs and the Department of Health for an out of court settlement of £42 million for 1217 haemophiliacs known to be infected with AIDS.

The Hepatitis C virus (HCV) was identified in 1989 and when a reliable test became available in 1991, the National Blood Authority screened donations. On 11 January 1995 the Department of Health announced that 3000 former hospital patients (survivors of an original total of more than 6000) who had received blood transfusions before September 1991 were being contacted, because a treatment was now available. On 30 January 1995 the Government rejected claims for compensation to be given to haemophiliacs who had contracted Hepatitis C from contaminated blood products.

HIV and AIDS in healthcare workers

Up to December 1995, of 79 reports of documented seroconversion after a specific occupational exposure, 46 were published in the USA and 4 in the UK. An additional 144 cases (8 in the UK) were possible examples of occupationally-acquired infection.[h]

It has been estimated that the risk of HIV transmission after a single percutaneous exposure was 0.32% and after a mucocutaneous exposure 0.03%.

The Expert Advisory Group on AIDS considered that most healthcare procedures posed no risk of HIV transmission and the risk of transmission from healthcare worker to patient was considered remote. Centers for Disease Control (CDC) in Atlanta reported transmission of HIV to patients during dental procedures carried out by a Florida dentist with AIDS, but the exact mode of transmission remained uncertain. All healthcare workers have an overriding ethical and legal duty to protect the health and safety of their patients, and workers infected with HIV must seek appropriate expert medical and occupational health advice. Exposure-prone procedures must cease and any physicians or occupational health practitioners, aware that infected workers had not sought or followed advice to modify their practice, should inform the appropriate regulatory body

2 *Nash v Eli Lilly* [1991] 2 Med LR 169

and the Director of Public Health of the district health authority in confidence.

Patients who have undergone an exposure-prone procedure during the preceding 10 years should be notified where practicable, face-to-face, by their family doctors or counsellors. The decision to undertake a lookback exercise should be made by the Director of Public Health after consultation with the UK Advisory Panel.[i] The General Medical Council has reaffirmed this advice on the duties of a doctor in October 1995.

Testing for HIV infection

Kennedy considered that both the criminal and the civil law, in particular the law relating to battery and the law relating to negligence, were relevant to the legality of testing.[j] A resolution at the 1987 Annual Representative Meeting of the British Medical Association (BMA) that doctors could, at their discretion, test patients without consent was not implemented, because the BMA Council was advised that doctors might take illegal action, and the 1988 Meeting resolved that testing should only be performed on clinical grounds and with the patient's specific consent.[k] The General Medical Council supports this advice.

HIV transmission and the law

In June 1992 there was national publicity[l] about an infected haemophiliac, who was believed to have slept with and infected several women, one of whom had died aged 20 of an AIDS-related illness in May. Arnheim[m] suggested criminal charges that could be brought: indecent assault (as in the Bennett case of 1866)[3]; assault occasioning actual bodily harm; and procurement of sex with a woman by false pretences. It is reported that action under the Offences Against the Person Act 1861, on the grounds of assault causing bodily harm, was considered and rejected. The patient denied the allegations, claimed he had not been counselled, and died aged 26 in Queen Elizabeth Hospital, Birmingham on 27 May 1994.

AIDS and homosexuality

Under the Sexual Offences Act 1967 the age of homosexual consent was set at 21. Society's attitude had altered radically since the

---

3 Rv Bennett [1866] 4 F and F 1105

Wolfenden Report of 1957 but an amendment to the Criminal Justice Bill to reduce the age to 16, thus making it the same as for heterosexuals, which was supported by the Health Education Authority, the British Medical Association and voluntary bodies, was lost in the Commons on 21 February 1994, an amendment to adopt the age of 18 was passed and the amended Criminal Justice and Public Order Act 1994 received the Royal Assent on 3 November.

AIDS and drug misuse

In 1988 there were estimated to be 75 000–150 000 injecting drug users, with an increased risk of HIV infection. The Third Report of the working party on AIDS and drug misuse[n] reviewed strategy in the period 1988–1993 and found that needle and syringe exchange schemes had substantially reduced the percentage of drug injectors sharing equipment from 60–70% in the mid 1980s to 21–38% in 1989/90.

Among the recommendations to the Prison Health Care Directorate were the wider practice of methadone detoxification for opiate addicts on reception, and making methadone treatment available for the longer term for those remanded or with short sentences. There should be confidential but easy access to condoms and decontaminants. The threats of transmission of Hepatitis B and C and HIV infection by drug users in prison in Australia (1991/92) and Scotland (1993) have been reviewed and the opportunities for prevention discussed.[o]

SUMMARY

The projections of AIDS incidence, mortality, prevalence and the number of persons with other severe HIV disease are set out in Table 15.1

Effective health education and a modification of lifestyles by homosexual and bisexual males, together with safe blood products and effective screening of blood donors, has reduced the risk of infection (see Fig. 15.1). Ante and intra-partum zidovudine has reduced the chance of maternal-infant HIV transmission by approximately two thirds.[p]

Aids cases and deaths by exposure category and date of report in the United Kingdom to 31 December 1995 are set out in Table 15.2.

Table 15.3 gives the geographical distribution of AIDS cases and deaths at 31 December 1995.

Table 15.1 Projections of AIDS incidence, mortality, prevalence, and the number of persons with other severe HIV disease (adjusted for underreporting). Source: Public Health Laboratory Service 1996, Communicable Disease Report Review, 1996; 1; 6 PRIS © PHLS

Year	AIDS* New cases (incidence)	Deaths	Cases alive at year end (prevalence)	Other severe HIV disease* Persons alive at year end and requiring care[†] (prevalence)
1994	1780	1570	3210	3210
1995	1950	1680	3485	3485
1996	2000	1790	3690	3690
1997	2025	1870	3845	3845
1998	2025	1925	3945	3945
1999	2010	1950	4010	4010

* Includes cases in children as well as adults.
[†] Prevalent AIDS cases multiplied by 1.

As Table 15.4 indicates, the United Kingdom has a more favourable experience than many other European Community (EC) countries. AIDS cases listed were reported to WHO by EC countries: cumulative totals at 31 December 1993.

In 1994, countries with the highest rates were, in descending order, Spain (185.2 cases per million population); Italy (99.1 per

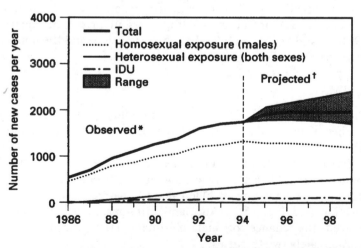

* Adjusted for reporting delay and 13% underreporting
†Adjusted for 13% underreporting

Figure 15.1 Observed (1986–94) and projected (1995–99) annual incidence of AIDS (England and Wales, data to end 1994)

Table 15.2 AIDS cases and deaths by exposure category and date of report: United Kingdom to 31 December 1995. Source: Communicable Disease Report 1996; 6: 25

How HIV infection was probably acquired	Jan 94 – Dec 94		Jan 95 – Dec 95		Jan 82 – Dec 95			
	Male	Female	Male	Female	Male	(Deaths)	Female	(Deaths)
Sexual intercourse between men[1]	1178	–	994	–	8617	6124	–	–
between men and women								
exposure to 'high risk' partner(s)[2]	8	22	4	29	41	24	133	83
exposure abroad[3]	140	98	117	119	705	398	505	253
exposure in the UK[4]	19	18	10	10	79	52	69	49
investigation continuing/closed[5]	7	3	16	6	29	9	9	2
Injecting drug use (IDU)	109	39	79	37	493	327	212	130
Blood factor treatment (e.g. for haemophilia)	70	–	100	–	554	488	6	5
Blood/tissue transfer (e.g. transfusion) abroad/UK	4	6	5	5	42	28	72	48
Mother to infant	23	23	17	17	88	48	94	45
Other or investigation continuing/closed[5]	12	2	10	9	102	77	22	11
Total	1570	211	1352	232	10750	7575	1122	626

1 Includes 196 men who had also injected drugs.
2 Partner(s) exposed to HIV infection through sexual intercourse between men, IDU, blood factor treatment or blood/tissue transfer.
3 Individuals from abroad, and individuals from the UK who had lived or visited abroad, for whom there is no evidence of 'high risk' partners.
4 No evidence of 'high risk' partners.
5 Closed – no further information available.

Table 15.3 Geographical distribution of AIDS cases and deaths by date of report: to 31 December 1995. Source: CDSC AIDS and HIV-1 Infection in the United Kingdom: monthly report. Communicable Diseases Report 1966; 5; p. 26

Country or region of first report	Jan 94 – Dec 94		Jan 95 – Dec 95		Jan 82 – Dec 95	
	Cases	(Deaths[1])	Cases	(Deaths[1])	Cases	(Deaths[1])
England						
Northern and Yorkshire	56	31	43	17	446	334
Trent	70	37	41	19	282	213
Anglia and Oxford	68	31	76	27	497	347
North Thames	929	371	795	139	6427	4184
South Thames	289	152	259	77	1854	1324
South and West	90	55	95	45	565	441
West Midlands	46	25	47	14	296	214
North West	79	38	62	23	548	420
Wales	23	16	20	11	160	137
Northern Ireland	7	2	13	5	62	44
Scotland	124	73	133	47	735	543
United Kingdom total	1781	831	1584	424	11872	8201
Ch. Islands/Isle of Man	–	–	–	–	6	5

1 These deaths are of patients referred to in previous column and known to have occurred at any time up to 31 December 1995.

million); France (98.1 per million). Although these three countries comprise less than half of the EC population, they accounted for more than three quarters of the AIDS cases diagnosed in 1994.[q]

Table 15.4 AIDS cases reported to WHO by EC countries: cumulative totals at 31 December 1993. Source: European Centre for the Epidemiological Monitoring of AIDS.

Country	Number of cases	Cumulative cases/million population
Spain	22655	579.4
France	28497	481.2
Denmark	1356	260.8
Italy	20336	351.8
Netherlands	2912	187.9
Germany*	10858	133.9
Belgium	1555	154.0
Luxembourg	77	192.5
UK	8529	147.1
Portugal	1641	167.4
Ireland	378	105.0
Greece	891	84.9

* Includes the former East Germany.

REFERENCES

a   Centers for Disease Control 1981 Morbidity and Mortality Weekly Report
    30:250. Pneumocystis pneumonia — Los Angeles. Centers for Disease Control,
    Atlanta
b   Centers for Disease Control 1981 Morbidity and Mortality Weekly Report
    30:305. Kaposi's sarcoma and Pneumocystis Pneumonia among Homosexual
    men — New York City and California. Centers for Disease Control, Atlanta
c   Communicable Disease Surveillance Centre 1994 Communicable disease report
    42:99. Communicable Disease Surveillance Centre, London
d   Communicable Disease Surveillance Centre 1995 Communicable disease report
    5:13. Communicable Disease Surveillance Centre, London
e   McCormick A 1993 The Times, 11 August
f   Dyer C 1987 Doctors with AIDS and the 'News of the World'. British Medical
    Journal 295: 1339
g   British Medical Journal Legal Correspondent 1985 Detaining patients with
    AIDS: British Medical Journal 291: 1102
h   Heptonstall J, Porter K, Gill N 1995 Occupational transmission of HIV.
    Summary of published reports. Communicable Disease Surveillance Centre,
    London
i   UK Health Departments 1994 AIDS/HIV-infected health care workers: guid-
    ance on the management of infected health care workers. Recommendations of
    the Expert Advisory Group on AIDS. HMSO, London
j   Kennedy I 1989 Testing for HIV infection: the legal framework. The Law
    Society's Gazette 86:30
k   Curtis H 1989 AIDS, health care and the law. The AIDS Letter, Royal Society of
    Medicine: 1:5
l   The Guardian 24 June 1992: At large with a lethal weapon
m   Arnheim M 1992: Three charges could be brought against an HIV carrier who
    infects others. The Guardian, 24 June 1992
n   Advisory Council on the Misuse of Drugs 1993 AIDS and Drug Misuse Update.
    HMSO, London
o   Gill O N, Noone A, Heptonstall J 1995 Imprisonment, injecting drug use and
    blood borne viruses. British Medical Journal 310:275–276
p   Connor E M, Sperling R S, Gelber R et al 1994 Reduction of maternal–infant
    transmission of HIV-1 with zidovudine treatment. New England Journal of
    Medicine 331:1173–1180
q   European Centre for the Epidemiological Monitoring of AIDS 1995 HIV/AIDS
    surveillance in the European Community and COST countries. Third Quarterly
    Report 1995. WHO-EC Collaborating Centre on AIDS, Saint-Maurice

16. Clinical trials: ethical, legal and practical considerations

Christobel Saunders

INTRODUCTION

Much basic medical research is carried out in laboratories. However, new diagnostic and therapeutic measures eventually need to be tested on humans — first by studying drug delivery and toxicity in healthy volunteers, then drug efficacy and activity in a limited group of patients — Phase I and Phase II studies. Following these studies a new treatment must be tested against conventional therapy by means of the Phase III study or randomized controlled clinical trial (RCT).

The RCT was first developed by RA Fisher in the 1920s for agricultural research, and was introduced some 20 years later into medicine in a trial evaluating antibiotic treatment for tuberculosis.[a] An RCT is a study in which a cohort of subjects with a defined disease are randomly allocated to one or other treatment (which may be an established versus either a new treatment, or using a placebo drug as the control) and their outcomes recorded. Randomization aims to avoid the types of bias inherent in observational studies, such as confounding, which may result in apparent differences between treatment groups which do not in fact exist.

By recruiting large numbers of subjects to a trial the chance that the outcomes between the two arms will differ because of unequal distribution of risk factors becomes small. It is possible to calculate this probability — the p value.

If a trial is designed to encompass any patients with a given condition the results can be generalized to the prevention or treatment of the disease as a whole.

This chapter explores the ethical issues surrounding RCTs and suggests that participation in clinical trials is the *most* ethical way to treat a patient. Practical points regarding the conduct of clinical trials will be discussed, and suggestions made as to why increasing numbers of patients are now asking to participate in trials. Legal principles which affect clinical experimentation will be considered.

Ethical issues

Ethics provide a pathway of reasoning whereby a morally respectable and defensible position can be reached.[b] The main ethical consideration when conducting a clinical trial is the dilemma between the doctor's duty to his patient and his duty to research. A balance of benefit must be reached encompassing the patient's opportunity to exercise autonomy and the doctor's secondary duty to promote the general welfare of society and ensure future generations of patients receive the best possible treatment.

It can be argued that not only does the doctor have a duty to undertake research but that the patient also has a duty to participate in clinical trials, as his treatment is a result of previous patients' contribution to medical science.

Clinical trials raise a number of problems for both the 'trialist' (i.e. the doctor) and the 'subject' (i.e. the patient). A doctor who participates in research must always put the good of the individual patient above the pursuit of knowledge. The patient expects that his doctor will first and foremost protect and promote his welfare. Yet the clinician may be genuinely uncertain as to the best possible form of treatment and so wish to enter his patient in a trial. He must then randomize the patient's treatment and may use a placebo. Explaining these issues to the patient may weaken the doctor-patient relationship — so often based upon the belief that 'the doctor knows best'.

If a patient does agree to enter a clinical trial it must be without coercion. In practice this may be hard to achieve as many patients feel they must agree to anything to 'please the doctor'.

These issues, along with the need to obtain informed consent, take on a portentous ethical and legal significance in the setting of a trial, leading some authors even to suggest that clinical trials are unethical.[c]

International guidelines

The attention of the medical community, and indeed the world, was first focused on the issue of the ethics of human experimentation following the disclosure of Nazi practices during World War II. In 1946, at the trial of 23 German doctors charged with 'war crimes' and 'crimes against humanity' for their experimentation on prisoners of war and civilians, the Nuremberg Code was established.[d] This aimed to protect the interests of human participants in research. Building upon this, the World Medical Assembly in 1964 adopted the Declaration of Helsinki containing 'recommendations guiding physicians in biomedical research involving human subjects'.[e] This has been updated, most recently in 1989.[f]

These guidelines recommend that a patient should firstly be assured of the best proven diagnostic or therapeutic method, and that any new treatment being tested will be *at least* as advantageous as any other, with a reasonably low chance of side-effects. The patient must be informed of the benefits and hazards of all possible treatments, and must be free to refuse to participate in a trial or withdraw at any time. The physician must also be free to change to another treatment if he feels this will benefit the patient. The patient may also anticipate that the doctor/investigator will keep any excess investigations in the trial to a minimum.

In the UK there is no statutory legislation on human experimentation (except the Human Fertilization and Embryology Act 1990). However, a number of medical bodies have developed their own guidelines. These include the Medical Research Council (MRC), the Royal College of Physicians, the Kings Fund, the British Medical Association, the Medical Sterile Products Association and the Association of the British Pharmaceutical Industry (ABPI).

Consent

To allow a patient to express his autonomy, he must be fully informed about his disease and its treatment. This will include details of the clinical trial he is being requested to join, along with the risks and benefits of all possible treatments (of course a patient outside a trial should also be informed of all possible treatments and not only the one he is offered). If he then consents to the treatment or trial this may be said to be informed consent (see also Ch.4).

The MRC in its 1986 document 'Responsibility in investigations on human subjects' states that: 'in general, patients participating in RCTs should be told frankly that different procedures are being assessed and their cooperation invited. Occasionally, however, to do so is contraindicated.[g]

Thus we are faced with another dilemma — although it is ethically imperative to obtain a patient's fully informed consent before initiating any treatment within a clinical trial, it appears that there may be situations in which full disclosure is harmful to the patient.[h] This predicament has been shown to be a major factor in poor accrual rates into clinical trials.[i]

Are RCTs ethical?

Faced with the twin dilemmas of trying to improve medical treatment using clinical trials yet not compromising an individual's right to choose his own treatment, and keeping a patient fully informed whilst not inflicting harm from overburdening him with data, one may wonder whether clinical research can ever be ethically sound.

As long as these issues are openly debated by all interested parties, then treating a willing patient within the context of a clinical trial is likely to satisfy the need both to offer the patient the best available treatment, and to improve our current treatments. In fact it has repeatedly been shown that the outcome of patients treated within a clinical trial is superior, no matter to which arm of the trial the patient is allocated.[j]

It is thus reasonable to argue that in the appropriate situation, offering a patient participation in an RCT is the *most* ethical treatment.

Legal issues

The Medicines Act 1968 regulates approval of all new drugs (See Ch. 14). If a pharmaceutical company wishes to use an unlicensed drug in a clinical trial they must usually obtain a Clinical Trials Certificate (CTC). A doctor (or dentist) must obtain an exemption (DDX provision) if he is using an unlicensed drug in an independent trial.

However in the UK there is no legislation specifically governing the conduct of clinical trials either of drugs or medical and surgical therapies. Some countries have enacted fuller legislation; for example the USA,[k] Australia, Eire, Germany, France and Spain. The situation in this country is not static, however, and the law slowly changes to reflect changing society.

Legal discussion regarding clinical trials, as well as standard treatment, has mainly centred around the issue of consent. Lord Scarman has said, 'If a patient is fit to receive information and wishes to receive it, the doctor must "brief" the patient so he can make a free and informed choice'.[1]

How much information should be given to the patient to allow him to make an informed choice, however, is open to interpretation and thus dissension. From an ethical standpoint there is a spectrum of views, ranging from those whose first concern is patient autonomy and full disclosure to those who adopt a paternalistic viewpoint in which the doctor must judge how much information he feels his patient requires, depending upon factors such as personality and perceived ability to understand information, the nature of the treatment and the magnitude of possible harm.

It is the latter view which has so far guided legal debate on this issue in this country, although the two cases which have been brought have concerned conventional treatment rather than treatment within a clinical trial.[1,2]

If a patient feels he has suffered harm as a result of being subjected to a treatment he may choose to bring charges of negligence or battery. He must prove that the doctor failed to provide sufficient information regarding the treatment and that this failure has caused him harm as he would not have consented to the treatment if full information had been given.

In the first case, *Bolam v Friern Hospital*,[1] the patient claimed he was subjected to electroconvulsive therapy (ECT) without relaxants or restraints and was not warned of the possibility of bone injury — he sustained fractures of the pelvis. It was found that failure to disclose this minimal risk was not negligent.

In the second case, *Sidaway v Governors of Bethlem Royal Hospital*,[2] again the plaintiff complained that she was not given sufficient information on the side-effects of her treatment, which she subsequently suffered, to allow her properly to consent to it. It was found that her doctor had acted in line with a 'reasonable body of medical opinion' as the risk of developing this side-effect was less than 1%, and so in this particular case was not negligent. These cases illustrate how the 'prudent doctor' is able to determine how much information a patient can be given.

Thus it would seem that in the absence of deliberate deception leading to the taking of unjustifiable risks or denial of an improved prospect of cure, action based on lack of consent is unlikely to succeed.

---

1 *Bolam v Friern Hospital Management Committee* [1957] 2 All ER 118
2 *Sidaway v Governors of Bethlem Royal Hospital and the Maudsley Hospital* [1985] 1 All ER 643

Many feel that the current state of the law fails to reflect full patient autonomy, although as Kennedy confirms,[c] there is in fact no law relating directly to clinical trials, as cases such as Sidaway concern treatment rather than experiment.

In the case of healthy volunteers in drug trials, the Association of the British Pharmaceutical Industry has issued guidelines concerning compensation.[m] The Consumer Protection Act 1987 states that a pharmaceutical company is liable for compensation for injury caused by a defective drug, and most pharmaceutical company sponsored trials will offer ex-gratia compensation schemes. However it can be contested,[n,o] that there is a need for some form of no-fault compensation procedure in all clinical trials, irrespective of whether or not they are run by a drug company, so that the burden of proving causation does not fall on the patient. This could be incorporated into the written consent form for participants in clinical trials.

It should be the responsibility of ethics committees who review research protocols to ensure this compensation is allowed for.

What is the likely outcome today for a patient who feels he has not been properly informed of some aspect of his treatment within a clinical trial? Kennedy[c] suggests that the courts would try to ensure that a patient had given informed consent and would use the doctor's evidence for this. If a doctor felt he had a compelling reason *not* to disclose fully all information this would almost certainly be accepted as being in the patient's best interests. It is accepted that there must be disclosure to a patient that he is in a clinical trial, and a doctor must answer honestly any questions posed to him by the patient: in giving permission for a trial treatment the patient does not surrender his rights and privileges. Furthermore: 'Even if a certain risk is a mere possibility that ordinarily need not be disclosed, yet if its occurrence raises serious consequences, as for example paralysis or even death, it should be regarded as a material risk requiring disclosure'.[3]

There are many questions which remain to be answered by the courts, the medical profession and patients. The question remains as to whether further moves towards increasing patient autonomy would eventually lead to a US-style system of full disclosure and exhaustive consent. If this happened, would it inevitably result in the practice of defensive medicine? If so, would the trust enshrined in the doctor-patient relationship be damaged by confusing and

---

3 *Reibl* v *Hughes* [1980] 114 DLR (3d) 1

worrying the patient with remote risks and technical details? Or is medical paternalism alive and well in the UK, bolstered by the judiciary, and set to stay?

Practical considerations

To be ethically and legally sound a clinical trial protocol must be based upon solid scientific design and good clinical practice. It must be performed by an experienced investigator and must have undergone review by an independent ethics (and preferably scientific) committee. Both the Department of Health and the Royal College of Physicians have made recommendations regarding the structure and function of ethics committees.[p,q]

A trial, whether run by a pharmaceutical company or a research institution, must be regularly monitored by an independent body to ensure that there is no misconduct, and that one arm of the study is not prematurely showing a significant beneficial or harmful outcome.

The investigator must ensure he obtains fully informed consent, preferably in written form, although there is no legal requirement in the UK for this and a witnessed oral consent may suffice. Such a consent should include the purpose of the trial, the benefits both to the patient and to society, any possible risks and alternative treatments, and the right to refuse or withdraw at any time. The patient should understand that results of the trial will be published, although he may be reassured that confidentiality will not be breached. The concepts of uncertainty and randomization should be explained.

It is important that patients are not coerced into entering trials; thus payment should not be offered in treatment trials, and healthy volunteers may only be paid a relatively modest sum. The use of 'captive audiences' in trials — such as medical students or prisoners — is somewhat controversial, although it may be said that any patient asked to enter a clinical trial by the doctor treating him feels under some obligation to comply to please the doctor.

The way forward

Is the goal of achieving certainty via the RCT too high a price to pay in ethical terms? Should we perhaps concentrate further on obtaining data from observational studies and other methods?

This author believes that well conducted randomized clinical trials continue to provide the best quality of data and offer the patient a fair plan of treatment. This can be further improved by good communication between the health workers and the patient including the use of counsellors, written information and interactive videos. Involving patients in the organisation of clinical trials and educating them to demand the best treatment, including treatment within a trial, should go hand in hand with educating doctors at undergraduate and postgraduate levels about the ethical, legal and practical issues involved in research.

Although the ethics of clinical experimentation have been widely debated, the legal standpoint awaits clarification until suitable cases have been brought to the courts.

Perhaps it would be reasonable to conclude that the consequences, both ethical and practical, of not performing proper randomized controlled clinical trials are too alarming to contemplate.

REFERENCES

a   British Medical Journal (author anonymous) 1948 Streptomycin treatment of pulmonary tuberculosis: a Medical Research Council investigation. British Medical Journal ii: 769–782
b   Ward C M 1994 Ethics in surgery. Annals of the Royal College of Surgeons of England 76: 223–227
c   Kennedy I 1988 Consent and randomized clinical trials. In: Kennedy I 1988 Treat me right. Clarendon Press, Oxford
d   US Government 1949 Trials of war criminals before the Nuremberg military tribunal under Control Council law; 2(10): 181–182. US Government Printing Office, Washington, DC
e   World Medical Assembly 1964 Declaration of Helsinki. Recommendations guiding medical doctors in biomedical research involving human subjects. Adopted by the 18th World Medical Assembly, Helsinki, Finland 1964
f   World Medical Assembly 1989 Declaration of Helsinki, amended by the 41st World Medical Assembly, Hong Kong, September 1989
g   Medical Research Council 1986 Responsibilities in investigations on human subjects. Medical Research Council, London
h   Saunders C M, Baum M, Haughton J 1994 Consent, research and the doctor-patient relationship. In: Gillon R (ed) Principles of health care ethics. Wiley, Chichester
i   Taylor K M, Margolese R G, Soskoline C L 1984 Physicians' reasons for not entering eligible patients in a randomized clinical trial of surgery for breast cancer. New England Journal of Medicine 310: 1363–1367
j   Stiller C A 1989 Survival of patients with cancer. British Medical Journal 199: 1058–1059
k   Department of Health and Human Services 1983 Title 45; Code of Federal Regulations, Part 46: revised as of March 8 1983. Department of Health and Human Services, Washington, DC
l   Scarman L 1986 Consent, communication and responsibility. Journal of the Royal Society of Medicine 79: 697–700

m   Association of the British Pharmaceutical Industry 1988 Guidelines for medical experiments in non-patient human volunteers. Association of the British Pharmaceutical Industry, London

n   Brazier M 1992 Medicine, patients and the law, 2nd edn. Penguin, London

o   Mason J K, McCall Smith A 1991 Law and medical ethics, 4th edn. Butterworths, London

p   Department of Health 1991 Local research ethics committees. HSG(91)5. Department of Health, London

q   Royal College of Physicians 1990 Research involving patients: 7: 86. Royal College of Physicians, London

Index